Rogue Cells

Rogue Cells

A Conversation on the Myths and Mysteries of Cancer

Richard J. Jones, MD,
and T. Michael McCormick, MS Ed

JOHNS HOPKINS UNIVERSITY PRESS | *Baltimore*

Note to the Reader: This book is not meant to substitute for medical care, and treatment should not be based solely on its contents. Instead, treatment must be developed in a dialogue between the individual and their physician. This book has been written to help with that dialogue.

© 2024 Richard J. Jones and T. Michael McCormick
All rights reserved. Published 2024
Printed in the United States of America on acid-free paper
9 8 7 6 5 4 3 2 1

Johns Hopkins University Press
2715 North Charles Street
Baltimore, Maryland 21218
www.press.jhu.edu

Library of Congress Cataloging-in-Publication Data is available.

A catalog record for this book is available from the British Library.

ISBN 978-1-4214-4828-2 (hardcover)
ISBN 978-1-4214-4829-9 (ebook)

Special discounts are available for bulk purchases of this book. For more information, please contact Special Sales at specialsales@jh.edu.

CONTENTS

Introduction

WHY ANOTHER BOOK ON CANCER, particularly by the two of us?

We decided to write this book together for several reasons. My boyhood friend of nearly 60 years, Dr. Richard Jones—a.k.a. Rick, for the balance of this book—had something important to say about cancer to a larger audience. I was interested in learning more about cancer the disease and, being recently retired, thought that I could help with the project.

Over our long friendship, many of our family members and friends have been touched by cancer. All of our parents died from cancer. My father was diagnosed with bile duct cancer and died a month later. My mother's lung cancer was a surprise diagnosis found through x-rays after she broke her hip in a fall. With our love and support, she suffered through two rounds of radiation therapy and went on to live five more happy and healthy years. Rick's father died of chronic myeloid leukemia (CML), which was universally fatal in the 1970s, when he was diagnosed. (Over the past 25 years, CML has become one of the real cancer success stories, with fatalities now uncommon.) Rick's mother died of pancreatic cancer that, like my mom's cancer, was undoubtedly related to smoking.

For much of our youth, Rick and I lived down the street from one another in a suburb near Harrisburg, Pennsylvania. We played on the same baseball teams and spent most of our summers together with our friends Steve, Bob, and Randy. We would hang out at the local public pool, play pickup sports (volleyball, wiffle ball, and football), and compete for endless hours in the three Ps (ping pong, pool, and pinochle). We'd listen to music (the Beatles, Simon and Garfunkel, Motown, and the occasional classical piece) and a few times got into trouble together. Although we hadn't planned it this way, we ended up attending the same college, Bucknell. Rick attended because it was the Jones family tradition (his dad, his brother, and later his son all went there); I went because I was interested in the best small liberal arts college in central Pennsylvania.

I've had many occasions to ask for help in dealing with cancer. My wife was diagnosed with lymphoma, and abdominal surgery was recommended. Luckily, Rick helped us figure out that she neither had lymphoma nor required surgery. In this and countless other instances, Rick has helped my family and friends understand the confusing flood of information that flows around cancer diagnoses and treatments, ask the right questions, and make the right decisions. Through these discussions, he has generously shared the knowledge and perspective that he has acquired in more than 35 years as a professor of oncology and medicine and as the director of the Hematologic Malignancies and Bone Marrow Transplantation Program at Johns Hopkins Medicine.

Rick had always—at least, for as long as I have known him—wanted to be a doctor. After four years at Bucknell studying biology and chemistry (and playing cards), he went to Philadelphia for medical

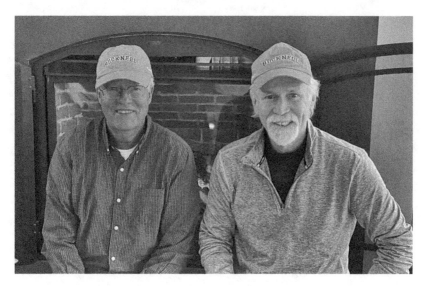

Rick (*left*) and Mike (*right*) in their Bucknell hats.

school at Temple University. Upon completing a residency in internal medicine, he got his first gig as a doctor at a family practice in central Pennsylvania. This specialty was a requirement of the Public Health Service scholarship he'd received for medical school. His choice of an oncology (cancer) fellowship at Johns Hopkins Medicine in Baltimore occurred after, and no doubt because of, his father's death from cancer. When his oncology fellowship ended in 1987, Rick decided to stay at Hopkins, where he has enjoyed a blended role of teaching, research, and patient care.

Over the years, I suspected that Rick was becoming well respected in his field because several times a year he traveled all over the world to speak at medical conferences and symposiums. Throughout this book, you will learn more about what Rick and his team have contributed to cancer research. Two highlights are their pioneering research into the cells that start cancer (cancer stem cells) and advances to eliminate the requirement for "perfectly" matched bone marrow (also called stem cell) donors.

Rick is a good teacher at Hopkins because he expects a lot of his students, as I can attest from his stern and knowledgeable advice on how to play pinochle better so we don't lose money to Bob and Randy and how to earn more master points in duplicate bridge. I've heard from his colleagues that Rick has a good bedside manner and helps his patients with a great deal of empathy. I know this to be true from the immense gratitude I've witnessed from family and friends whom he has helped.

So Rick is clearly qualified to write this book. What about me? If Rick could be said to have had a laser focus on a medical career, my career focus was blurry at best. After applying to music schools, I started out majoring in math and then rapidly shifted to liberal arts when math turned too abstract. This allowed me to take a wide spectrum of courses, mostly in the humanities, and I majored in religion and philosophy. What did I do with a religion major? I was drafted into the Army, where I served for two years as a Pershing missile crewman in Germany; worked as a children's services caseworker assisting low-income families; got a master's degree in educational research and school psychology; worked for two years as a county human services planner; and finally found my niche in the emerging computer and software field.

After all of the above, here's what I bring to this book on cancer designed for laypeople: (1) I knew little about the subject to start with, so if I could understand it enough to accurately get it down on paper, then there is a good chance that others would understand it as well; (2) I saw the toll that cancer could take, both emotionally and physically; and (3) I like to understand how things work, asking probing questions like, How much do you think that tree weighs?

As a researcher and teacher, Rick has frequently told me that his most important job is educating his students and his patients about the science of cancer. For patients, his hope is that, with a better understanding of simple cancer biology, they will become full partners in the management of their disease instead of being limited by fear of their diagnoses. Rick's approach to educating students and patients involves coming up with stories and anecdotes that make the biology of cancer more approachable for the non-expert.

As we began to discuss this project, our primary goal was to make cancer as comprehensible as possible. We thought that Rick's scientific background, experience, and stories (you'll learn a lot about dandelions and their roots, and about flies, lightning, and Singapore) combined with my being relatively uninformed on the topic would work well. Our challenge was to make cancer understandable to a wide audience while accurately capturing the current state of knowledge in this rapidly changing field of medicine. The book is a true collaborative effort (there will be no Lennon and McCartney bickering about who wrote what), but we decided to write the book under one voice—mine, as the naive layperson—to enhance clarity.

Understanding the causes of cancer and discovering new treatments is complex. Physicians and researchers have been trying to answer these questions for centuries, and they are still trying. Cancer is as old as humankind, and although much has been learned, much has yet to be understood. In this book, we will attempt to cover topics in enough detail to build a general foundation for understanding cancer. We also provide helpful references for digging deeper into the specifics. We've written the text to make science as "unsciencey" as possible, but for those who want to delve a little deeper into the science and biology of certain individual topics, we've provided "Science Corner" sidebars to answer some of your questions.

Our goals for this book are to

- help you better understand what is known and not yet known about cancer biology, prevention, and treatment;

- debunk some of the myths that surround the disease;
- enable you to ask good questions and make informed decisions with the help of your physicians, family, and friends; and
- most importantly, approach cancer with more hope and less worry and fear.

Rick and I enjoyed writing this book together. We hope that you enjoy it as well, and learn something, too. I know I learned a lot.

CHAPTER 1

Cancer's Myths and Mysteries

CANCER WILL INEVITABLY TOUCH YOUR LIFE. You or someone close to you—a family member or a friend—will be diagnosed with cancer. You will have lots of questions. What kind of cancer is it? When did it start? What caused it? Why? What is the best treatment? Is it curable? How long do I have to live? In this book, we provide information about cancer and its treatment so that the answers to these questions will be more understandable. Early on in our book discussions, Rick shared these highlights with me:

- Cancer is not uniformly fatal, and two-thirds of people diagnosed with cancer now survive five years and longer.
- Many cancers are slow growing and often don't even have to be treated.
- Although many cancers are not curable, they become more like chronic diseases, such as high blood pressure and diabetes, which require treatment but with which you can live a long life.

- An increasing number of cancers are considered curable, although we still have a long way to go on this front.

I used to be scared of cancer, but then it really grew on me

Rick tells me he likes to start lectures with a joke to loosen up both the audience and himself. He believes that maintaining a sense of humor is key to a healthy approach to dealing with cancer for patients and families as well as their doctors. My friends with cancer affirm this belief. The section heading above—Rick's favorite cancer joke, told to him by one of his patients—drives home the need for a sense of humor even when dealing with something as scary as cancer. Rick actually wanted to subtitle the book "How I learned to stop worrying and not fear cancer," based on the tagline of the movie *Dr. Strangelove*. This 1964 dark comedy about another scary topic of not so long ago, the Cold War and the atomic bomb, is one of Rick's favorite movies. In addition to interjecting some humor, this movie reference was meant to highlight a major objective of this book: making cancer a little less frightening. So, if you are wondering why we think *Dr. Strangelove* is relevant to a nonfiction book on cancer, skip ahead to chapter 11 or enjoy the suspense.

I agree with the need for humor when dealing with such a serious topic, but all joking aside, the bullet points above may not alleviate one's fear. When Rick first showed me these bullet points, here were my initial reactions:

- So, if I get cancer tomorrow, I will have a 33% chance of dying within five years.
- I don't particularly like the idea of cancer growing in me and, even if no treatment is recommended, having to wait for it to get worse.

- I've lived with high blood pressure for most of my adult life, but there is a little tiny pill that I can take every day to keep it in check.
- It's reassuring that more cancers are considered curable; I just hope I get one of those.

Now, having written this book, I can understand Rick's excitement about the progress that these points reflect. I hope that by the end of the book you will feel the same and that we have presented a convincing argument for accepting cancer as part of life and not fearing it.

Cancer in a nutshell

In the simplest terms, cancer is a disease caused by the growth and spread of cells that are not well behaved. Cancer cells grow too much, fail to die when they are supposed to, and spread to unwelcome places. Most cancers are caused by errors that occur when normal cells divide and multiply. These errors are called mutations: random changes to the structure of a gene within a cell that are passed onto future cells within the cancer. The occurrence of genetic errors during cell division is a natural process that happens tens of billions of times every day. The body does a pretty good job of cleaning up random mutations—but not a perfect job. Is it just bad luck at the cell division poker table that random mutations become cancer? The answer isn't fully understood, but there are three other important influences on whether mutations become cancer: environmental agents, inherited genes, and the body's natural defenses.

Our environment can expose us to known cancer-causing agents, or carcinogens. These agents damage cells, causing mutations and increasing the risk of cancer. For example, the chemicals in tobacco smoke are known to cause lung and other forms of cancer. As cigarette smoking has decreased in the United States since the 1970s, there has been a marked decrease in lung cancer. Other carcinogens have also been identified, such as asbestos, which is associated with mesothelioma and other cancers, and exposure to ultraviolet sunlight, which is linked to a higher incidence of skin cancer. The evidence is fairly weak for many other environmental agents that have been popularly characterized as carcinogens; more on that later.

Most cancer-causing mutations are acquired—they are not present in the person at birth. Certain cancers, however, have been shown to be linked to inherited cell mutations—that is, genetic defects that are passed down in the family. A few rare inherited genetic mutations almost always lead to cancer; most do not. For most inherited genetic mutations, like *BRCA1* and *BRCA2* (BReast CAncer gene, pronounced "bracka"), there is simply an increased chance of getting cancer.

While links have been established between cancer and both environmental agents and inherited genetic mutations, neither one alone actually causes cancer. We have all heard about the 95-year-old, cancer-free chain smoker. Keeping with our poker analogy, a "bad cancer deal" can happen for several reasons: some players get drunk at the table and as a consequence misplay the hand (environment), some players are genetically predisposed to be poor poker players (heredity), and it is a game of chance (luck), after all.

The role of the body's natural defenses in both preventing cancer and slowing its growth is a hot research topic. Our bodies' immune systems, which defend against infections, likely hold part of the explanation for why some people get cancer and some don't. The immune system is a potent anticancer agent, and medical science is just learning how to harness it to treat and cure cancer. If you've seen any television commercials lately, you've likely heard about all the new immunotherapies—treatments that boost the body's immunity to fight cancer.

Is cancer becoming more prevalent? Yes, if you think wrinkles and gray hair are more common.

While cancer isn't spreading like the flu usually does in the winter, or as COVID-19 was in 2020–21, the number of people living with a cancer diagnosis has never been greater. In fact, 40% of individuals will get cancer during their lifetime. Cancer has nearly caught, and will likely soon overtake, heart disease as the number-one cause of death in the United States. There are several reasons for this increase, but none are because cancer is contagious, as was once thought to be the case. In the 1600s two doctors in Holland, Zacutus Lusitanus and Nicolaes Tulp, reached this conclusion based on their experiences with breast cancer in members of the same household. They proposed that cancer patients should be "isolated, preferably outside of cities and towns, in order to prevent the spread of cancer."

Cancer is increasing because people are living longer and not dying of other ailments, like infections and heart disease. Cancer is an age-related disease: the incidence increases as individuals grow older, especially after age 60. If one lives long enough, one will likely develop cancer. In fact, more than 90% of those diagnosed with cancer and who die of cancer are over the age of 50.

Over the past 160 years, life expectancy from birth in the United States has risen from 39.4 years in 1860 to 78.9 years in 2020. Just since 1960, life expectancy for both men and women has increased by roughly 10 years (figure 1.1). For many people, cancer is a part of aging, along with increased aches and pains, wrinkles, and gray hair. And like the tree that falls in the forest that no one hears, many people will die from other causes without ever knowing that they had cancer.

Cancer isn't just a single disease. There are innumerable types of cancer, each with unique characteristics. Virtually every organ in the body can develop cancer. Historically, oncologists treated all cancers

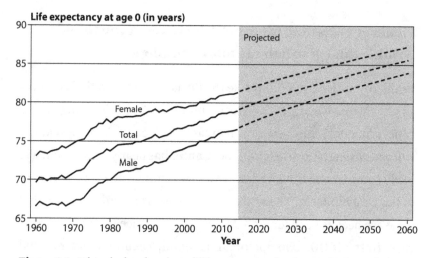

Figure 1.1. Historical and projected life expectancy for the total US population at birth, 1960–2060. Over the past 160 years, life expectancy in the United States has risen from 39.4 years in 1860 to 78.9 years in 2020. Just since 1960, the life expectancy for both men and women has increased by roughly 10 years. (*Source:* US Census Bureau, 2017 National Population Projections, 1960–2060; and National Center for Health Statistics Life Tables, 1960–2014, https://www.cdc.gov/nchs/data/nvsr/nvsr68/nvsr68_07-508.pdf.)

from the same organ similarly: all patients with lung cancer got the same treatment, as did all patients with breast cancer or leukemia. We now know that within each organ-specific cancer, there are scores to hundreds of different cancer types, each of which requires a somewhat different therapy, often based on the cancer's unique genetic mutations. Some cancers, such as myelodysplastic syndrome (MDS), weren't even classified as cancers until recently (see the Science Corner on MDS for more information about this "new" cancer).

Another reason for the apparent increased incidence of cancers is completely artificial. Today we are much better at diagnosing cancers than we were in the past. Many cancers are now identified at a much earlier stage through screenings and early detection strategies, such as Pap tests for cervical cancer, CT scans for lung cancer,

SCIENCE CORNER

Myelodysplastic Syndrome

Myelodysplastic syndrome (MDS) was not classified by cancer registries like the National Cancer Institute's Surveillance, Epidemiology, and End Results (SEER) Program until this millennium. MDS is a sometimes (but not always) serious form of leukemia that was once called preleukemia even though cancer researchers have known for decades it is actually a blood cancer. The cancer starts in a blood stem cell that continues to make mature but often malformed blood cells, at least for a while. Like leukemia, lung cancer, breast cancer, and all broad cancer types, there are many different forms of MDS. In serious forms of MDS, the disease eventually stops making the blood cells and acts like acute leukemia.

MDS is rare in patients under age 50, but it is becoming epidemic in older patients—a prime example of cancer's association with aging. Other cancers have also only recently been identified through advances in cellular biology and genetics.

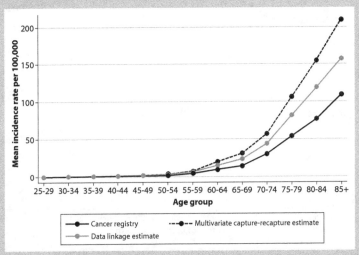

Estimate of MDS incidence, 2003–2010. The solid black line is the reported incidence, but MDS is underreported owing to difficulties in diagnosis before the advent of molecular testing in the past decade. The dashed line represents the statistical estimate of actual incidence. (**Source:** Reprinted with permission from McQuilten ZK et al., Underestimation of myelodysplastic syndrome incidence by cancer registries: results from a population-based data linkage study, *Cancer,* 2014; 120(11):1686–1694.)

mammograms for breast cancer, colonoscopies for colon cancer, and PSA blood tests for prostate cancer. Predictably, with the widespread introduction of these screening and early detection strategies in the second half of the twentieth century, new cancer case rates rose rapidly between 1975 and 1990 (figure 1.2). The fact that since about 1990 cancer rates have plateaued or even decreased confirms that the increase in the last quarter of the twentieth century represented improved detection methodologies.

Even though more cancer is being diagnosed, the cancer death rate over the past 40 years has declined by more than 25% (figure 1.2).

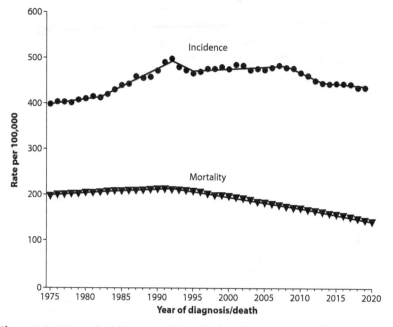

Figure 1.2. Cancer incidence over time. There was a rapid increase in new cancer case rates between 1975 and 1990 with the widespread introduction of cancer screening and early detection strategies in the second half of the twentieth century. Since about 1990, however, new cancer rates have plateaued or even decreased, confirming that the increase in the last quarter of the twentieth century represented improved detection methodologies. Despite more cancer being diagnosed, the cancer death rate has declined by more than 25%. (*Source:* SEER Program, National Cancer Institute. Incidence data are from the SEER 9 areas.)

This progress has been made possible by both earlier diagnosis and big improvements in treatment options, which we discuss in chapters 7 and 8. What is even more encouraging in these numbers is that cancer deaths in the past were underreported. Many deaths were attributed to "natural causes" or "old age." Now an actual cause of death is more often identified.

Is cancer preventable? Well, yes and no . . .

Rick has a simple answer: cancer as a broad classification of diseases is not preventable. At times we all probably stress about what we can do to lessen our chances of getting cancer (figure 1.3). Let me put your mind at ease: while lots of laboratory studies suggest stress can cause changes that may affect cancer growth, there is no clinical evidence that stress truly causes cancer. There is also no evidence that any combination of dos or don'ts is the silver bullet to prevent all types of cancer. If we live long enough, some form of cancer is likely. Still, there is no question that for many cancers, such as lung cancer and cervical cancer, certain actions will greatly reduce a person's risk.

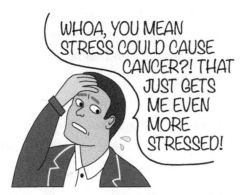

Figure 1.3. The good news is that despite some data in the laboratory showing that stress can trigger chemicals that affect cancer cell growth, there are no clinical data showing that stress causes or influences cancer growth.

Most approaches to reducing the risk of cancer focus on the following behaviors:

- Don't use tobacco.
- Eat a healthy diet.
- Maintain a healthy weight and be physically active.
- Remove asbestos and radon gas from buildings.
- Protect yourself from the sun and ultraviolet radiation (don't use tanning beds).
- Find precancerous conditions early (get your Pap tests and colonoscopies).
- Get immunized to prevent infections that can lead to cancer (such as human papillomavirus, or HPV, and hepatitis).

What is the life expectancy for someone with cancer? Better than you might expect.

I gained some important insights into what a diagnosis of cancer really means when my mom was diagnosed with lung cancer. Although my mom was a long-term smoker, her diagnosis at age 80 still came as a shock. Her lung cancer was incurable, and my mom and all the family feared the worst. Nevertheless, she lived five quite normal years after the diagnosis, playing lots of golf and enjoying her family and friends up until the very end.

Survival rates differ depending on the type of cancer and the stage of the cancer when it is diagnosed. The National Cancer Institute's Surveillance, Epidemiology, and End Results (SEER) Program has collected and shared a wealth of data on cancer trends in the United States since 1975. Some people live a long time with cancer. Results for all types of cancer show survival rates of about 70% at

5 years and 50% at 30 years. Women diagnosed with breast cancer have about a 90% survival rate at 5 years and an 85% survival rate at 10 years. These numbers have been steadily improving for the past 40 years.

While population-wide trends for survival with cancer give reason to hope for a long life with cancer, each individual's experience with cancer is unique. It is impossible to provide a specific answer to the question, How long will I live? Statistics aren't prescriptive, and overall probabilities can't predict an individual outcome. You can't predict a single coin toss of heads or tails based on a 50% probability of heads across lots of coin tosses. Longevity, even for a single type of cancer, can vary. Some people die within the first year, while others with the same cancer are still alive after 30 years. I will discuss the reasons for these differences later.

The fact that many people are living longer with cancer changes everything. Since cancer is often no longer an imminent death sentence and a call to get your life in order, the focus shifts to balancing treatment options, minimizing symptoms, and staying healthy and active.

Improvements in treatments over the past several decades have enabled a better quality of life both during and after treatment. In general terms, treatments are

- more targeted, causing less damage to healthy cells;
- better controlled, causing fewer and less debilitating side effects;
- leveraging the body's natural immunities and getting the body to fight back; and
- keeping people healthier by focusing on nutrition, exercise, rest, and so on.

Through advances in treatment, an increasing number of cancers are now considered curable. Most patients with aggressive lymphomas, for example, can now expect to be cured. Despite this encouraging data, the term "cure" is becoming less relevant in relation to many forms of cancer. In the past, living five years without a recurrence of cancer was considered a cure; now, however, we know many cancers can remain dormant for years and even decades. While surviving five years after a cancer diagnosis is certainly a desirable milestone, eliminating the recurrence of life-threatening cancers—the true definition of "cure"—is most desirable, even in patients in their 60s and 70s, who could otherwise expect to live another two to three decades.

We now know that many cancers are slow growing, or indolent, and relatively well behaved for decades. These indolent cancers can be thought of as similar to high blood pressure, which, while incurable, is not a death sentence if appropriately monitored and treated.

Are we winning the war on cancer? Again, yes and no . . .

The "war on cancer" has been a rallying cry to raise money, fund grants, and mobilize research to fight cancer for decades. Many regard the National Cancer Act, signed into law by President Richard Nixon in 1971, as the beginning of the war on cancer. This legislation supported the US commitment to fighting cancer, which in 1970 was the nation's second leading cause of death. The bill strengthened the National Cancer Institute (NCI), which had been established in 1937 by President Franklin Roosevelt, by giving the director authority to plan and develop a National Cancer Program that included the NCI, other research institutes, and other federal and nonfederal programs. It also created NCI-Designated Cancer Centers (figure 1.4).

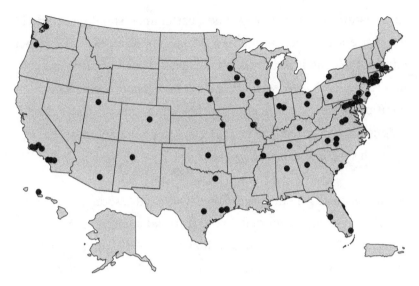

NCI-Designated Cancer Centers

The 71 NCI-Designated Cancer Centers are at the forefront of NCI-supported efforts at universities and cancer research centers across the United States. The centers are developing and translating scientific knowledge from promising laboratory discoveries into new treatments for cancer patients. There are 13 cancer centers, 51 comprehensive cancer centers, and 7 basic laboratory cancer centers.

Figure 1.4. NCI-Designated Cancer Centers, which were established by the National Cancer Act of 1971. (*Source:* National Cancer Institute, NCI-Designated Cancer Centers, 2019, cancer.gov/cancer-centers.)

As a campaign, the war on cancer has been effective. Funding and resources have been mobilized, progress has been made, and many battles have been won. While it is fair to say we are winning the war, it is more accurate to say that the war on cancer isn't really winnable. Cancer is an inevitable result of natural processes in our bodies. The war on cancer should be considered part of the ongoing struggle to live longer and healthier lives.

Today, fighting cancer is arguably an even greater priority than it was in 1971. Research over the past several decades has dramatically improved our understanding of cancer. We have identified the genetic markers or mutations underpinning most cancers, gaining critical information on cancer biology and a better understanding of individual cancers and their prognoses. Most important, our new knowledge of the genetic mutations that cause cancer provides targets for new therapies that are setting the stage for big improvements in treatment outcomes. Identification of these mutations is also aiding in diagnosis, and possibly even true early detection, of many cancers through simple blood tests.

In this chapter's general discussion, I have tried to scratch the surface on what is known about cancer and dispel some myths that surround it. While improvements in lifestyle—most significantly, fewer smokers—have reduced cancer, this decline has been offset by increases in cancer diagnoses as people live longer. There is no way to prevent most cancers, although healthy lifestyle choices can delay its development. Earlier diagnosis through effective screenings and improved treatments mean that people are living longer and healthier lives. In the following chapters, we will explore all of these aspects in more detail. I hope you enjoy the journey.

CHAPTER 2

Cancer Biology

Cells Going Rogue

IN THE NEXT TWO CHAPTERS, I will review the basics of cancer biology, which will serve as the backdrop for the rest of the book. In the simplest terms, cancer is a disease caused by the growth and spread of normal cells that are no longer well behaved—they've gone rogue. Normal cells become cancer as a consequence of errors, called mutations, that develop in the genes of these cells. A gene is a section of the chromosome that provides valuable information for how a cell functions (see the Science Corner on normal cell biology).

In general, the mutations that cause cancer occur in the genes that regulate and control normal cell growth and survival. While normal genes do a respectable job of ensuring orderly and controlled cell growth, mutated genes cause "dysregulated" (a fancy word for "not at all controlled") growth. Think of watching a five-year-old's soccer match. To make matters worse, these dysregulated cancerous cells are clonal: the mutations in one cell are passed down to all the cells in the cancer, so now all the cells grow abnormally. Cancer-causing mutations can result from (1) environmental toxins (such as cigarette smoke), (2) hereditary predispositions, or (3) random errors in cell division that occur naturally.

SCIENCE CORNER

Normal Cell Biology: Understanding the "Biological Atom"

The human body is an amazing machine. However, even the best machines eventually stop working properly. To figure out why any machine is malfunctioning, one first needs to understand how it normally operates. So, before discussing how cancer disrupts the workings of this amazing machine, I'm going to explain the biology of normal cells. By combining our backgrounds (science in Rick's case and nonscience in my case), we hope to make this explanation more understandable than most owner's manuals.

Cells, trillions of them, are the basic building blocks of this machine we call the human body. Cells combine to form the tissues or organs (for this discussion I'll use these terms interchangeably) that keep the machine functioning. Calling cells "building blocks" is an imperfect analogy. Perhaps a more appropriate one was coined by the English philosopher George Henry Lewes, probably better known as the common-law husband of Mary Ann Evans (pen name: George Eliot): "A cell is regarded as the true biological atom." Atoms combine to form molecules, and molecules combine to form all the matter or substances that make up the universe.

There are two broad types of cells: gametes and somatic cells. In the simplest terms, gametes, or germ cells (sperm and eggs), are responsible for reproduction, and somatic cells (from the Greek word for body: *soma*) make up everything else: bone cells, muscle cells, nerve cells, blood cells, and so on. There is no standard classification for different cell types in the body, but the most commonly quoted number for different types of somatic cells is 220. However, the number of different cell types could easily go up depending on how much of a lumper or splitter you are.

Just as some atoms, like hydrogen, can function on their own, so can some cells, such as the red blood cells that carry oxygen throughout the body. Other cell types combine to form organs, often with different types of cells. For example, the skin (or epidermis) is an organ made up of four types of cells.

Like atoms, cells are active, with many moving parts. Cells take in nutrients from the food we eat and convert those nutrients into energy to carry out specialized functions. Cells also contain the body's hereditary material, allowing them to make copies of themselves (or undergo cell division) as needed for the body to grow and to repair damage.

Each cell normally contains 23 pairs of chromosomes. A chromosome is made up of proteins and deoxyribonucleic acid (DNA) organized into genes. A human is estimated to have between 80,000 and 100,000 genes, all made up of different sequences of DNA. Every cell contains all the same genes, such that each and every cell contains all the genetic instructions needed for the entire body. Through complex chemistry (for me, magic), genes are turned "on" or "off" depending on the needs and function of the specific cell so that a heart cell looks and acts like a heart cell and a blood cell looks and acts like a blood cell. For more information on genes and how they are turned on or off, see the Science Corner on DNA and RNA.

SCIENCE CORNER

DNA and RNA

Each of the 46 chromosomes (23 from each parent) contains hundreds to thousands of genes, the basic physical and functional unit of heredity. Genes contain the instructions for the development and function of living things. Every person inherits one gene from each parent and thus has two copies of each gene. Most genes are the same in all people, but a small number of genes (less than 1% of the total) are slightly different between people. These minor differences contribute to each person's unique physical features.

Genes are a short segment of deoxyribonucleic acid (DNA), which occurs as a fine, corkscrew-shaped thread (or helix) that coils around like a twisted ladder. Genes vary in size from a few hundred DNA bases to more than 2 million. The DNA strands are the side rails, made from alternating phosphate and sugar groups, and the rungs are the four molecules (adenine, cytosine, guanine, and thymine—called

(continued)

nucleobases, or bases for short) that provide all the instructions needed for cell function and replication. The human genome consists of approximately 3 billion base pairs of DNA.

An important property of DNA is that it can replicate, or make copies of, itself. Both strands of double-stranded DNA store the same biological information, so each strand of DNA in the double helix can serve as a pattern for duplicating the sequence of bases. This is critical when cells divide because each new cell needs to have an exact copy of the DNA present in the old cell. That is a lot of information to duplicate correctly every time! Less than 2% of the DNA, or about 20,000 genes, actually code for the proteins that carry out the cells' heavy lifting. In other words, these genes provide instructions for the proteins that support cell growth, communication with other cells, and even cell death. Gene regulation—that is, what turns DNA on or off in a specific cell so only those genes needed by that cell are active—is the result of changes that do not affect the DNA sequence. Chemical compounds are added to single genes to regulate the gene's activity; these modifications, called epigenetic changes, are critical to why a heart cell looks and acts like a heart cell and why a brain cell looks and acts like a brain cell.

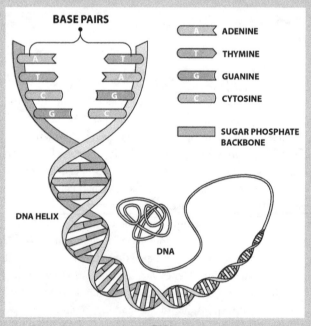

DNA

If the DNA genes are the lead actors in our cancer plot, then RNAs are the strong supporting actors. RNA stands for ribonucleic acid, and its primary role is to convert the information stored in DNA into proteins. Messenger (m)RNA (of COVID-19 vaccine fame) carries the protein blueprint from a cell's DNA to its ribosomes, which are the cellular protein factories. Regulatory RNA constitutes the factory quality assurance specialists, which limit the amount of mRNA that is produced and regulate the production of proteins from mRNA (a process called translation). The function of a vast majority of the cell's genome (DNA) is currently unknown.

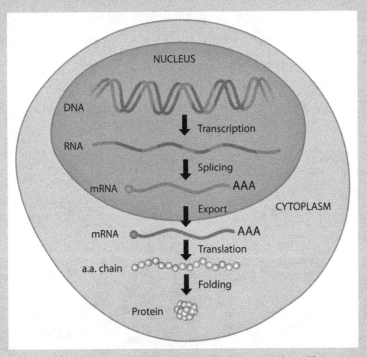

Transcription and translation. AAA = adenine; a.a. = amino acid.

Environmental toxins: Smoke and errors

All of us are familiar with several environmental toxins that have been linked to cancer-causing mutations. Many probably think that environmental toxins cause most cancers. Doctors have known for years that cigarette smoking greatly increases the risks for not only lung cancer but also cancers throughout the body (figure 2.1). The poisons in cigarette smoke and other tobacco products can damage a cell's DNA, causing mutations. And these poisons can weaken the body's immune system, making it harder to kill cancer cells. Outside of tobacco, however, environmental toxins appear to play a minor role in cancer causation.

Certain viruses have also been linked to cancer-causing mutations. We are putting viruses in the "environmental toxin" bucket

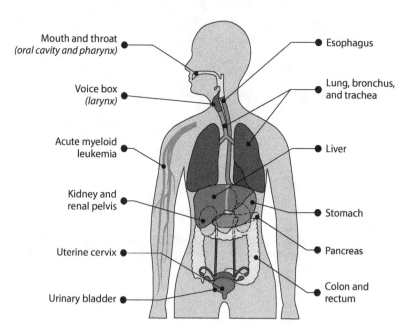

Figure 2.1. Tobacco use causes many different types of cancer. The American Cancer Society estimates that smoking causes about 20% of all cancers and about 30% of all cancer deaths in the United States.

because viruses come from external sources and they travel through the body acting like a toxin—doing harm and triggering the body's immune system. When viruses cause an infection, they spread their DNA or RNA, affecting healthy cells' genetic makeup and potentially causing them to turn into cancer. Two prime examples of potential cancer-causing viruses are the Epstein-Barr virus (EBV), which leads to infectious mononucleosis, and the human papillomavirus (HPV).

So far, there have been more than half a billion cases of COVID-19 worldwide, leading to over a million deaths in the United States alone. The COVID-19 virus can hit the body hard, affecting not just the respiratory system but also the heart, brain, and kidneys. During the COVID-19 pandemic it was important to protect existing cancer patients, who were at greater risk owing to their compromised immunity, mostly as a result of treatment. Will COVID-19 illness later result in cancers? Rick says it is too early to ask this question. To date, none of the coronaviruses, which were first identified in the 1960s, are known to increase the risk of cancer.

It is difficult to estimate the share of cancer that is triggered by environmental toxins. The US Centers for Disease Control and Prevention have estimated that up to 15% of cancers seen today can be prevented by avoiding unhealthy environments and lifestyles, especially smoking. The role of environmental toxins in causing cancer will be discussed in more depth in chapters 9 and 10.

Hereditary predisposition: It's not really your parents' fault

Some people are born with mutations inherited from their parents, such as the *BRCA* mutations associated with a higher risk of breast, ovarian, and other cancers. Mutations in specific genes are associated with more than 50 hereditary disorders that may predispose individuals to developing certain cancers. The National Cancer Institute estimates, however, that inherited genetic mutations play a significant role in only about 5%–10% of all cancers (figure 2.2).

Doctors often recommend genetic tests when someone has a strong family history of cancer or when clinical findings suggest an inherited cause of cancer. Inherited predispositions to cancer are genetic mutations passed from parent to child that often lead to cancer, typically at a younger age than usual for that cancer type. However, inherited genetic predispositions are not uniformly harmful, since it almost always takes more than one mutation to cause cancer, as will be discussed in a bit. Unfortunately, many of the inherited genes that predispose people to cancer also appear to interfere with the repair of damaged DNA, making additional mutations more likely. But don't blame your parents—it is likely that natural selection

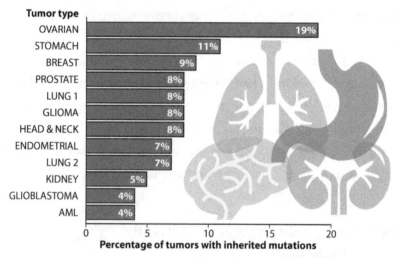

Figure 2.2. Cancers associated with inherited mutations. Lung 1 = squamous cell carcinoma; lung 2 = adenocarcinoma; AML = acute myeloid leukemia. (*Source:* Used with permission from Washington University School of Medicine / Sara Moser, based on data from Lu C et al., Patterns and functional implications of rare germline variants across 12 cancer types, *Nat Commun*, 2015 Dec. 22;6:10086.)

failed to eliminate inherited genetic predispositions to cancer because they provided an evolutionary advantage early in life.

SCIENCE CORNER

Inherited Cancer Genes

Cancers linked to inherited genetic mutations include the following:

- inherited breast and ovarian cancers (*BRCA1* or *BRCA2*)
- Lynch syndrome (hereditary non-polyposis colorectal cancer)
- Li-Fraumeni syndrome (rare familial syndrome associated with many different cancers and caused by inherited mutations in the *TP53* gene)

It appears that inherited cancer syndromes were not eliminated through natural selection because they provided an evolutionary advantage early in life. Such an advantage would allow individuals with the mutation to have a better chance of surviving through childhood and into child-bearing years, even though it would ultimately increase the risk of cancer later in life.

Perhaps the best-understood example of such an evolutionary advantage is the ability of the inherited gene mutation that causes sickle cell anemia to provide protection against malaria. Malaria attacks red blood cells, and individuals in Africa and around the Mediterranean who carried the sickle cell trait (that is, one sickle cell gene) had a survival advantage when infected with malaria, over those with normal hemoglobin. As most of the world has eliminated malaria, the survival advantage of sickle cell trait has also been eliminated, and all that is left is the harmful effects in individuals with two sickle cell genes (those with sickle cell anemia).

Scientists have theories about what evolutionary advantages other inherited genetic cancer predispositions may have provided to individuals to allow them to survive through their child-bearing years. However, we will likely never know for sure as most of these health risks—such as malaria, which was historically fatal in childhood—have been eliminated.

Random errors in cell division: Mistakes are a part of being human

It is human nature to seek a cause for everything that happens to us, good or bad. For example, my mom always told me that going out in the cold with a wet head would make me sick. Even at a young age, Rick told me this wasn't true. Score one for Rick. Colds are caused by viruses, so you won't catch one from going outside with wet hair.

Increasing evidence suggests that most cancers do not have an external cause that can be prevented or avoided. Rather, most cancer-causing mutations appear to be random errors—or bad luck—as a natural consequence of the many normal cell divisions needed to keep us alive and healthy. If a person lives long enough, one of these unlucky cell divisions will likely occur and lead to cancer.

Why is this the case? We've all grown up thinking that cancer—more specifically, the mutations that cause cancer—is preventable if we can just figure out the cause, as was done for cigarette smoking and lung cancer. It turns out, however, that most of the random errors that cause cancer occur because the normal process of making new cells—cell division—is extraordinary and complex.

- First of all, the adult human body consists of more than 30 trillion (10^{12}) cells.
- Roughly a trillion cell divisions are needed every day to maintain and repair all the body's tissues and organs. Red blood cells are the dominant cell type, making up more than 70% of all cells in the body and accounting for an equivalent percentage of cell divisions.

- Taken together, more than a quadrillion (10^{15}) cell divisions occur over a person's lifetime (see the Science Corner on big numbers).
- Cell division copies all of the information coded in the genes of the original cell, moves the copied genes into a new cell, and then splits the cell. Each cell replication duplicates 3 billion (10^6) bits of information.

Given the complexity in accurately replicating all this information, we should probably be asking "how does cell division ever go right?" instead of "why does cell division sometimes go wrong"? Why isn't cancer more prevalent than it already is?

An exact gene mutation frequency—an error rate—during cell division is hard to pin down. Mutation rates are influenced both by the nature of the gene and by environmental factors. Best estimates are that more than a trillion mutations occur in a person's DNA daily. Most of these mutations have no ill effects, for a couple of reasons. First, there is a good chance that the genetic error will be in a part of the genome that does not affect the cell's growth and survival functions—good news. Second, the body's immune system is busy at work eliminating cells with mistakes—also good news. However, a mutation has a chance of avoiding the immune system's surveillance system—this is bad news, but it marks just the beginning of a long battle that may or may not ultimately result in cancer.

The bottom line is that the longer someone lives, the greater their chance of developing a cancer-causing mutation. Although it may not be possible to avoid cancer if an individual lives a long life, healthy living is an effective strategy for delaying cancer and living even longer. It should be possible to modify the relationship between age and dying from cancer.

SCIENCE CORNER

Big Numbers!

There are 30 trillion cells in the human body (plus or minus a few billion)

To put this number into perspective, you must think really big. How about the number of stars in the universe? You need 100 galaxies like our Milky Way, with between 100 and 400 billion stars in each galaxy, to get close to the 30 trillion cells in the human body. Through natural processes, these trillions of cells continually die and need to be replaced.

One trillion cell divisions occur every day to maintain the 30 trillion cells

Another way to visualize a colossal number like one trillion is to think in terms of time:

- There are 86,400 seconds in a day.
- A million seconds (1,000,000) is about 12 days—or how long a recent study found it takes parents to get fed up with their kids during summer vacation.
- A billion seconds (1,000,000,000) is 31 years—or how long it takes the typical self-made millionaire to get rich.
- A trillion (1,000,000,000,000 or 10^{12}) seconds is 31,688 years. If we went back that far in time, we would be at the end of the last ice age, when almost all of Canada and some of the northern United States were covered in ice.

More than a quadrillion cell divisions occur in a human life span

One trillion cell divisions a day × 365 days in a year × 80 years = 30 quadrillion, give or take a few. This number is beyond anyone's comprehension, but the figure will give you some idea.

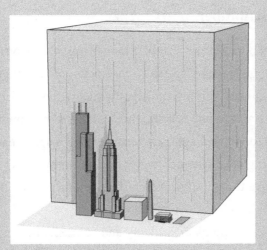

How big is a quadrillion? A stack of a quadrillion pennies compared to the Sears Tower (now the Willis Tower), the Empire State Building, a stack of a trillion pennies, the Washington Monument, the Lincoln Memorial, and a football field.

Each cell replication duplicates 3 billion bits of information

Cell division copies all the information coded in genes of the original cell, moves the copied genes onto a new cell, and then splits the cell in two. Each somatic cell has 46 chromosomes—23 contributed by the father and 23 by the mother. Each set of chromosomes contains 50,000 to 100,000 genes carrying a total of 3 billion base pairs, or bits of information—the complete set of cellular instructions. Duplicating all this information for a single cell is equivalent to the task of making 3,000 copies of every word in the seven books in the Harry Potter series by J. K. Rowling, which together contain roughly 1 million words.

So how many base pairs are duplicated in a lifetime?

Thirty quadrillion cell divisions in a lifetime × 3 billion base pairs = about 100 septillion (10^{26} or 100,000,000,000,000,000,000,000,000, 000). A stack of this many pennies would be more than a trillion times bigger than the one depicted in the figure. With so much copying going on, it should surprise no one that genetic mistakes are the norm.

Cancer cell numbers and Carl Sagan

If all these exponents and numbers in the "millions" haven't yet made your head spin, I must regretfully pose one more number challenge: How many cancer cells are there at diagnosis? The short answer is a lot. Cancer starts as one cell and must go through many replications before even sensitive diagnostic tests can pick it up. Size is important for diagnosing solid cancerous growths. Lung tumors, for example, must be larger than 5 millimeters (the size of a pencil eraser) before they are visible on x-rays or MRIs.

Rick asks his medical students and residents how many cancer cells are typically present at diagnosis, and they rarely if ever get the answer right. The most common answer given, he reports, is a million cells. In fact, the answer is between 100 billion and a trillion cells (figure 2.3). It is possible to pick up smaller cancers with very sensitive techniques, but even with the best technology available today, it is

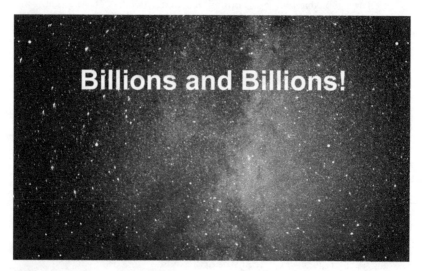

Figure 2.3. Famous quote attributed to Carl Sagan on the number of stars in the galaxy (or cells in a cancer at diagnosis).

virtually impossible to diagnose cancer before it has reached 100 million cells.

Depending on how fast the cells in a particular cancer divide, it can take a long time to replicate this many cancer cells. Since cancer is clonal—it starts in one cell—cancer cell growth can be thought of as a process of doubling. In other words, one cancer cell divides and becomes two, two cancer cells divide and become four, and so on. It takes about 30 doublings to reach a billion cancer cells. To prove this for yourself, use an exponential calculator app or search for one in your browser. Use logarithm base 2 to reflect that two cells are replicating, and watch the numbers grow.

To reach 100 billion to 1 trillion cancer cells, the point when most cancers can be diagnosed, requires between 35 and 40 doublings. At just over a trillion cells in size, cancer imposes a burden on the body that is usually fatal. Some patients get extremely sick and even die within a few weeks or months after they are diagnosed, leading friends and family to wonder how the cancer could grow so quickly. What they generally don't know is that 30 to 35 out of the 40 doublings (75%–88% of the cancer's life span) occurred before it was ever diagnosed.

The fastest-growing cancers, such as Burkitt lymphoma, double every 12 to 24 hours, so they may have been around for only a month or so before diagnosis. Most cancers, however, take weeks or months to double, and the slowest take years, which means that most patients have had cancer for years, or even decades, before it can be diagnosed. As an example of the lifespan of a typical cancer, figure 2.4 shows a cancer with a doubling time of 100 days. Forty doublings would take more than 10 years (100 days × 40 doublings = 4,000 days). Even using the best available detection means, the cancer would be completely undetectable for 8 years. If left untreated, it would be fatal in just 2 years—which would represent only 20% of its total life.

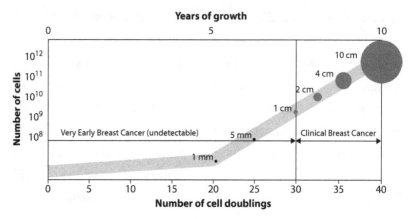

Figure 2.4. Life of a cancer with a doubling time of 100 days, which is a common doubling time for many solid tumors like breast cancer, prostate cancer, and colon cancer. The small number of cancer cells involved in the doubling initially makes it seem like the cancer is growing more slowly than it does once it's detected. Generally, cancers are undetectable until they reach about 100 million to 1 billion cells (more or less the size of a pencil eraser). Even using the best available detection means, the cancer would be completely undetectable for eight years and, if left untreated, would be fatal in just two years after detection—a period that in fact represents only 20% of its total life. Even though the doubling time of 100 days does not change, the large number of cancer cells involved in later doublings, once cancer is detectable, makes the cancer seem like it is growing faster.

The final crucial point related to cancer growth and diagnosis is the concept of cancer cell heterogeneity. Although all the cells in a cancer are related (arising from the same initial cell), they are no longer the same after 35–40 doublings. To illustrate, let's assume that all humans arose from a single person, and let's call that person Adam (or if you prefer, *Homo sapiens* #1). No two individuals look alike, think alike, or act alike, and there are only 8 billion of us. Even identical twins have slight differences. Now multiply 8 billion times 100, and you can imagine the diversity or heterogeneity of cells within a cancer. Cellular heterogeneity is a critical aspect of cancer's ability to progress as a disease and is a primary reason that not all therapies work on every cell in a cancer. I'll come back to cancer cell heterogeneity in a bit.

How do mutations cause cancer? Singapore and air conditioning

The number of cells in most organs and tissues are tightly controlled by mechanisms that, for the most part, maintain organ size and function throughout adult life. There are only three ways in which the cell numbers of an organ or tissue abnormally increase: (1) too many new cells are produced through cell division, (2) cells live too long, or (3) cells travel to the organ from somewhere else (for more information, see the Science Corners on tissue homeostasis and cell division).

Rick uses the small island city-state of Singapore to illustrate the three ways in which organ or tissue cell numbers would increase abnormally. In 1820 Singapore's population was about 1,000; today it is 6 million. How has it grown 6,000-fold in 200 years? In the mid-1800s, people from many areas, particularly China and Southeast Asia, migrated—or metastasized, if you will—and by 1900 the population exceeded 200,000. In the 1900s, particularly after World War II, Singapore saw a huge increase in population that was driven almost entirely by an increased birth rate and longer life expectancy. Between 1900 and 1950, Singapore's birth rate increased nearly 10-fold, bringing the island's population to 1 million in 1950. The median life expectancy has increased from about 45 years in 1900 to 83 years today. Cancer uses the same mechanisms for its accelerated growth: metastatic spread, overproduction, and prolonged survival.

There is one more component critical to the growth and development of cells, both normal and cancerous: the special environment that nurtures cells. Lee Kuan Yew is remembered as the man who transformed Singapore from an island with few natural resources when he took power in 1959 into one of the wealthiest countries in the world when he left power in 1990. When asked about the secret of Singapore's success, Lee highlighted the importance of tolerance

SCIENCE CORNER

Tissue Homeostasis

Cells of different types have different life spans. Red blood cells live for about four months. Some white blood cells (neutrophils or granulocytes) live hours to a few days, while other white blood cells (lymphocytes) live on average more than a year. Skin cells live for about two or three weeks. Colon cells die off after about four days. Sperm cells have a lifespan of only about three days, while brain cells typically last an entire lifetime (neurons in the cerebral cortex, for example, are not replaced when they die).

The life span of cancer cells is different from normal cells, and that is what often causes problems. Typically, cells die by either apoptosis (also called programmed cell death) or necrosis. In apoptosis, cells are shed without damage to the surrounding tissues, like leaves dropping in the fall. Necrosis is messier. Toxic materials seep out, uncontrolled, into the surrounding cells and tissues, causing even more damage.

Normal tissue growth and repair are regulated or controlled through processes that maintain homeostasis—that is, a steady, stable, and balanced state. For cells with shorter life spans, more frequent cell division is needed to maintain cell numbers. Different cell types have different pre-programmed life spans. At any given time, adult humans, for example, have roughly 20–30 trillion red blood cells, which is approximately 70% of all the cells in the human body by number. Given the relatively short life span of red blood cells, the body needs to make about 2 million new ones per second to keep up. Genes within each cell regulate growth (cell division) and cell survival or death. Cancer-causing mutations in genes can cause cells not only to grow too fast but also to live too long.

among different ethnic groups (the country has a Chinese majority with sizable Indian and Malay minorities). Surprisingly, the second factor he highlighted was air conditioning (figure 2.5), which provided the environment that made development possible in the tropics. Although there are no statistics on this topic, Singapore was

SCIENCE CORNER

Cell Division

For tissues to grow, new cells must be made. The process of making new cells is called cell division, and the cell cycle is the series of events that takes place in a dividing cell. The cell cycle is essentially the life span of the cell. The events that make up the cell cycle include the duplication or copying of the cell's DNA (DNA replication) and some of its organelles (or smaller cellular components), and subsequently the partitioning of its cytoplasm and other components into two daughter cells. Mistakes in the cell cycle, particularly during DNA replication, can lead to cancer. The steps in the process of cell division are as follows:

- usual day-to-day activities (first gap phase—G1)
- synthesis of chromosomes, proteins, and other molecules that are needed to replicate the second strand of DNA (synthesis phase—S)
- preparation to divide (second gap phase—G2)
- cell division (or mitosis—M)

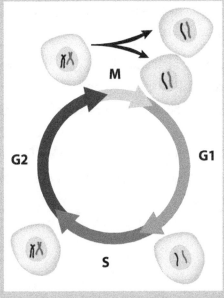

Cell division and the cell cycle.

At mitosis, the parent cell no longer exists but becomes two daughter cells. Sometimes the daughter cells are cloned copies of the parent—this so-called self-renewal is an essential characteristic of stem cells. Sometimes the daughter cells are slightly different and are no longer able to divide; in this case they just die rather than going through the cell cycle. This process is called senescence (from *senex*, the Latin word for "old") and is the fate of most somatic cells.

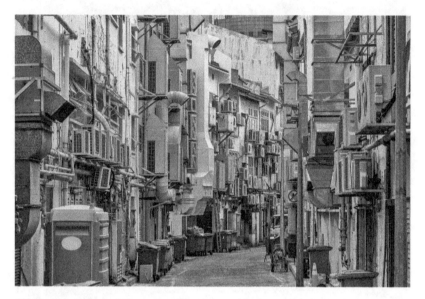

Figure 2.5. A typical Singapore side street, with air conditioners galore.

once called the most air-conditioned city in the world. It has now likely been surpassed by Houston and Dubai, two other hot cities whose rapid growth benefited from an air-conditioned environment. As will be discussed in more depth later, whenever a cancer grows by traveling from one place to another (metastasizing), producing too many cells, and living too long, it needs a favorable microenvironment to flourish.

CHAPTER 3

Cancer Stem Cells

The Dandelion Phenomenon

MOST OF YOU ARE FAMILIAR WITH the term "stem cell" but perhaps have never heard the term in relation to cancer. It turns out that understanding one particular type of stem cell, a cancer stem cell, is vital for fully understanding how cancer develops, grows, and behaves.

Stem cells: What's all the buzz about?

Most cells in the human body are differentiated—they are designed to carry out a specific function. Red blood cells, for instance, carry oxygen. It is helpful to think of each organ in the body as analogous to a beehive. Differentiated cells are the worker bees. Like the worker bees, differentiated cells (1) cannot reproduce; (2) do their various jobs (housekeeper, nurse or nanny, guard, forager, and so on); (3) die off (usually after only a month); and (4) are replaced by new worker bees.

There are two broad categories of cells in the body: germ cells, which are responsible for sexual reproduction, and somatic cells, which are all the other cells in the body. Stem cells are a class of somatic cells from which the other somatic cells originate or "stem." Although there is a lot of buzz concerning embryonic stem cells, the parents of all the cells in the body, those are only one small class of stem cells (figure 3.1). Every organ has a stem cell from which the rest of the organ develops. Accordingly, a stem cell (a queen bee, if you will) is the "parent" of the rest of the somatic cells—the "children" (worker bees) that constitute the bulk of the organs (hives) of our body. Unlike human parents (and queen bees for that matter), however, stem cells have the additional ability to clone themselves, or self-renew. This is the primary function that defines stem cells.

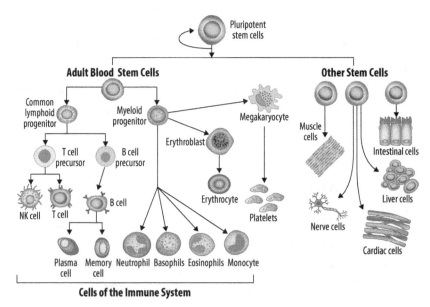

Figure 3.1. Different types of stem cells and their "children." Embryonic (pluripotent) stem cells are the parents of all the cells in the body. All the organ-specific (multipotent) stem cells, which are the parents of all cells within a specific organ, arise from the embryonic stem cells. (**Source:** Dipnarine Maharaj, South Florida Bone Marrow Stem Cell Transplant Institute.)

The first-discovered and best-understood organ stem cells are the blood stem cells, or hematopoietic stem cells (*hemato* = blood, *poietic* = to make), which are the parents of all the blood cells in the body. This big family of cells includes

- many different white blood cells that form the immune system responsible for protecting the body against infections;
- red blood cells that carry oxygen to the tissues; and
- platelets that help blood to clot.

Similarly, other adult organ stem cells produce distinct types of children. For example, the brain and nervous system stem cells produce two major cell types: (1) nerve cells or neurons, which transmit the nerve signals, and (2) glial cells, which provide support and protection for the neurons.

What happens when one of the differentiated cells comes to the end of its short life? Since all cells have the machinery to make more cells or replicate, it might make intuitive sense for the skin cell right next to a dead skin cell to get on with mitosis and fill the gap. But that would lead to cellular chaos, with every neighboring cell trying to jump in and help. In reality, differentiated cells, like skin and all other organ cells, rarely replicate. They are born, do their jobs, grow old, and die, like worker bees. In a hive, the task of controlling the hive's size is left to only one bee: the queen. Similarly, in an organ, the task of maintaining cell numbers and maintaining organ homeostasis is left up to one specialized cell: the organ stem cell. Leaving the task of tissue homeostasis up to one cell allows that cell to keep order. Stem cells are one of the smallest cells in an organ, but in this case, size doesn't matter—they still have all the genetic instructions needed. Stem cells are pretty wonderful, but if a stem cell gets confused, all heck can break loose, leading to cancer.

Another function of organ stem cells is their ability to travel throughout the blood to replenish and repair tissues. This ability seems fairly obvious for blood stem cells, but it is also how other adult stem cells repair their respective organs. It is hard to imagine stem cells traveling from one end of a solid organ to another to replenish an old or damaged cell, so it makes sense that they hitch a ride through the bloodstream. And their small size enables stem cells to move around the body to wherever they are needed to repair their respective organs.

Let me recap by going back to the simplest terms. Differentiated somatic cells are the building blocks of the body (like worker bees in the hives) while stem cells (like queen bees) are the long-lived factories for these cells, with the ability to travel throughout the blood when and where they are needed.

Continuing the parental analogy, there are many generations of stem cells, from parents to grandparents to great-grandparents. Embryonic stem cells can be thought of as Adam and Eve; they are the first parental cells of the entire person. They are called pluripotent (*pluri* = many, *potent* = having power), meaning they can produce all the cells in the body. In addition, every organ of the body has specific adult stem cells that can keep the organ functioning by replacing old or damaged cells with new ones. These stem cells are called multipotent because they can produce all the different cells in a specific organ, but not cells in other organs.

Adult organ stem cells share two other characteristics with queen bees: they are the longest-lived members of the organ (hive), and they are rare, hidden within the mix of their much more numerous children, which represent most of the members of the organ (hive) (figure 3.2). The rarity of stem cells has made them hard to find and learn about, but new techniques have recently made it much easier to hunt them down and study them.

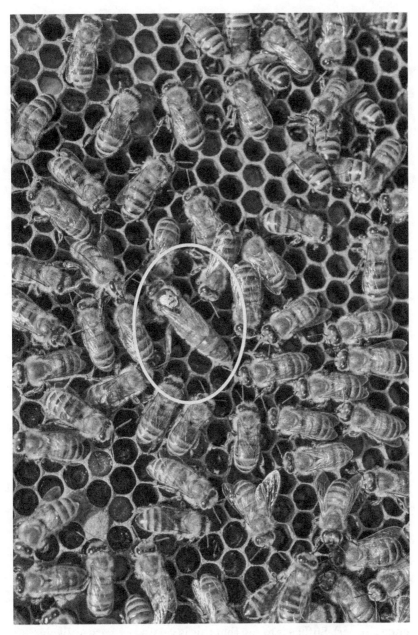

Figure 3.2. Like a queen bee hidden in the hive by all her worker bees, rare stem cells are hard to find among all the cells in an organ (or cancer).

Cancer stem cells: Getting to the root of the problem

Although there are nearly a trillion cells (more than 100 times the number of humans on Earth) present in a cancer when it is diagnosed, cancer starts in one cell. One mutation alone, however, almost never causes cancer—it usually takes at least three mutations, and often more. In the 1950s, several cancer researchers hypothesized that by the time of diagnosis most cancers have acquired three to seven mutations that drive the development of the cancer. As genetic research has become increasingly sophisticated during this millennium, researchers have confirmed this hypothesized number of "driver mutations." In actuality, most cancers have many more than seven genetic mutations (often hundreds) at diagnosis, but most are so-called passenger mutations—random consequences of the uncontrolled cell divisions, just along for the ride—and play little role in the cancer biology.

A cell destined to become cancerous must survive long enough to accumulate the three to seven genetic mutations necessary to fully generate the disease. Most somatic cells in the body are like the worker bees: they are neither long lived nor able to self-renew. Most normal cells live less than a year, and some live only a few days. Since normal somatic cells are unlikely to live long enough by chance to develop the exact three to seven genetic mutations required to drive cancer, they would need to develop them simultaneously or in rapid succession. Developing the three or more mutations needed to become cancer in cells living less than a year is like being hit by lightning three times in less than a year (see figure 3.3 and the mutational frequency Science Corner). Suffice it to say that this is very, very, very unlikely.

If you're like me, you may find it easiest to take it on faith that most normal cells don't live long enough to become cancerous. After my class in modern abstract algebra, with a textbook of 100 pages and not

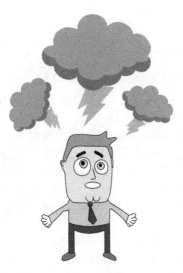

Figure 3.3. Lightning striking someone thrice in a year has never been reported. Similarly, it is unlikely that non-stem cells would acquire the multiple mutations that would cause cancer during their life span.

a single number, did me in, I quickly changed my college major from math to religion and philosophy. The philosopher in me prefers deep questions about how things work to mathematical proofs. So the next question excites me: if most normal cells do not live long enough to develop the three to seven mutations necessary to become cancer, how then do normal cells go fully rogue?

At least a half a century ago, researchers hypothesized that the inherent longevity and extensive proliferative capacity of an adult organ stem cell make it an ideal candidate to become a cancer-initiating cell. Studies in the laboratory were showing that the cells responsible for producing cancer in a petri dish or an animal were only a small fraction of the malignant cells, just as the queen bee is the only bee to reproduce in a hive. The findings reminded the researchers at the time of stem cells, so they called them cancer stem cells. Researchers back then lacked the tools to prove that cancer truly started in adult organ stem cells, and the concept fell out of favor for a quarter of a

SCIENCE CORNER

Mutational Frequency and Lightning Strikes

The mutation frequency associated with normal cell division is about 1 in 10,000—similar to the odds of being hit by lightning over one's lifetime. The odds of being hit by lightning a second time in the same year (again most non-stem cells live less than a year) are $10,000 \times 1,000,000$ (the chance of being hit by lightning in any one given year), and the odds of being hit a third time are $10,000 \times 1,000,000 \times 1,000,000$, or 1 in 10,000,000,000,000,000 (that's 1 in 10 quadrillion). Since there are only 30 trillion (30×10^{13}) cells in the body, the occurrence of three mutations simultaneously or in rapid succession in normal cells in the body is a virtual statistical impossibility. After all, if the chance of winning the lottery is a thousandfold lower than the number of players, it is unlikely that anyone will ever win.

century. With the development of more sophisticated laboratory techniques around the turn of the millennium, however, Rick and his research colleagues around the world were able to show that many, if not most, cancers started in adult organ stem cells. These cells are long lived—many are nearly immortal—giving them time to develop three to seven mutations over their lifespan, and they have the ability to produce more cells and propagate the cancer.

These relatively rare cancer stem cells are biologically different from the much more numerous cells (their cancer "children," if you will) that make up the bulk of the cancer. The cancer stem cells look and act differently from their cancer children, but they are also especially problematic because they maintain many of the characteristics of the adult organ stem cells from which they arose. Rick compares them to dandelions. The parts of the plant we can see—the stem, leaves, and flowers—are not what primarily keeps the dandelion hardy (figure 3.4). The root, which looks nothing like the rest of the weed,

SCIENCE CORNER

Multistep Process of Oncogenesis

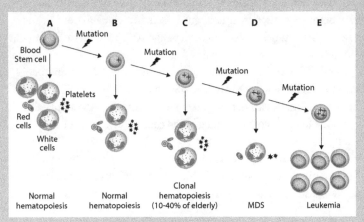

Multistep process of oncogenesis.

The figure above depicts the stepwise development of cancer, starting with normal blood stem cells and progressing through a series of mutations that eventually leads to myelodysplastic syndrome (MDS) and ultimately to full-blown leukemia. This multistep process, called oncogenesis (from the Greek: *onco* = tumor, *genesis* = production), occurs more or less in a similar fashion in all cancers. In this leukemia example of oncogenesis, normal blood stem cells produce all the cellular components of blood (*A*) in a process called hematopoiesis (keep it in mind if you find yourself with lots of vowels when playing Scrabble). Mutations will inevitably develop in dividing stem cells, but most of these mutations are of no consequence because they are in a part of the genome that does not affect the cell's function (*B*).

Eventually a random mutation could hit a hot spot—a part of the gene that does matter for cell growth and survival. One such mutation will usually not cause cancer, but it could give the stem cell a growth advantage over other similar stem cells. A blood stem cell developing a growth advantage is called clonal hematopoiesis, where the blood cells still behave normally but are dominated by those from one stem cell (*C*). In this case, blood cells, which normally come from many

(*continued*)

different stem cells and are thus not related, come from just one parent stem cell. Since the related blood cells are still normal, patients with clonal hematopoiesis are otherwise normal, and although they do have a slightly increased risk of developing leukemia, most never will. The incidence of clonal hematopoiesis increases with age: it is rare before age 40, occurs in about 10% of individuals over 60, and is present in most people who make it to age 100. Thus, in many ways, it can be considered a normal part of aging.

Additional mutations sometimes occur in the clonal hematopoiesis stem cells, leading to MDS. MDS, which used to be called preleukemia, is actually early-stage leukemia (D). Although the stem cells continue to produce functioning blood cells in MDS, they often look funny and their numbers are reduced, so people with MDS frequently require transfusions. Finally, additional mutations could eventually lead to full-blown leukemia, in which the blood cells produced by the leukemia stem cell are called "blasts" and no longer function at all (E).

does that heavy lifting. The root is hidden from view, like normal stem cells, which are rare and hard to find. If we try to get rid of the dandelions by removing just the visible part of the plant—by mowing the lawn, for instance—we'll be constantly thwarted in our attempts to keep them from growing back. In fact, cancer stem cells often look and act much more like normal stem cells than their cancer children. I wonder how many of us could distinguish a dandelion root from the root of any other weed or from a tulip. Even Rick's two-year-old grandson can distinguish a dandelion—he loves blowing the fuzzy white seed head and picking the pretty yellow flower—but he has never dug up the root to have a closer look.

Normal stem cells are the most resistant cells in the body to toxic insults like smoking, because they need to maintain the cellular reserve that can produce new cells for a person's life. This inherent resistance to toxic insults gets passed on to cancer stem cells and is one of the reasons they are relatively resistant to anticancer therapy. Can-

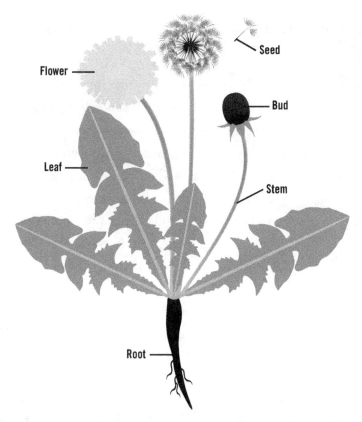

Flower

Seed

Leaf

Bud

Stem

Root

Figure 3.4. The dandelion phenomenon. Cancers, like dandelions, are heterogeneous. That is, cancers can have different-looking and different-acting cells (similar
to the flowers, leaves, and stems of the weed). This heterogeneity includes cancer
stem cells, which are hidden, are completely different from the rest of the cancer,
and need to be removed to eliminate the invader, just like the dandelion root.

cer stem cells also maintain the ability of normal stem cells to travel
through the blood to get to areas that need repair. These properties of
cancer stem cells have important implications for metastasis and treatment responses. Many cancer treatments are like mowing dandelions;
they don't remove the undetectable, biologically different (cancerous)
root. This is essentially why many treatments induce remission, but
the disease comes back. I'll discuss cancer stem cells and their implications for cancer biology and treatment in the following chapters.

Cancer mutations: One bad apple does not always spoil the whole bunch

A mutation can give cells within an organ a growth advantage and still not be cancerous. One mutation alone almost never causes cancer (figure 3.5) but instead usually provides a cell with a growth advantage that leads to benign—nonmalignant or noncancerous—growths. With the development of additional mutations, however, some of these changes in cells may eventually lead to cancer. In general, the difference between a benign lump and cancer is the lump's inability to invade and damage the organ or spread (metastasize). Three examples of growths or lumps that are not cancer are hyperplasia, dysplasia, and carcinoma in situ.

"Hyperplasia" is the term used when cells within an organ build up but the organ's structure remains normal and the cells still look

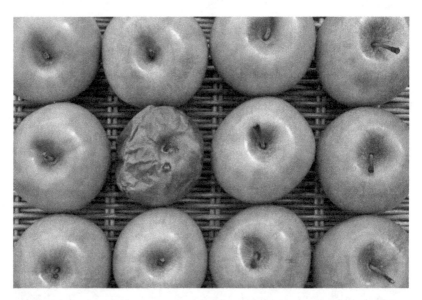

Figure 3.5. One bad apple did not spoil this whole bunch, just like one mutation almost never causes a cell to become cancer.

normal under a microscope. This is almost always the result of a genetic mutation in cells that makes them live too long but has no other effect on the cell's behavior. Hyperplasia can be caused by the same factors that induce the mutations that cause cancer, including chronic irritation, viruses, and just bad luck.

Common skin moles may be the most common form of benign hyperplasia. Most cases of the skin cancer melanoma start in a mole, but only rarely do moles become skin cancer. Usually, moles are just watched unless one begins to look funny. Colon polyps are another common type of hyperplasia. Since colon polyps are internal and can be observed only through colonoscopy, they are generally removed to prevent any chance that they will develop additional mutations and convert to colon cancer. Clonal hematopoiesis and monoclonal gammopathy of undetermined significance (MGUS) involving plasma cells are benign hyperplasias of blood cells. Since these cells circulate through the body in the bloodstream, they cannot be removed and are thus just watched.

These are just a few examples of hyperplasia; every organ in the body can have such benign growths. It is important to distinguish these from cancer because they are much more common than cancer, and every one of us will have at least one type—such as moles—if not several types of benign hyperplasia during our lifetimes.

Dysplasia is a more advanced condition than hyperplasia but still benign. In dysplasia, there is also a buildup of extra cells, but the cells look abnormal and there may be changes in how the organ is organized. In general, the more abnormal the cells and tissue look, the greater the chance that cancer will eventually develop. Some types of dysplasia need to be treated, while others do not. Perhaps the most common example of dysplasia is an abnormal skin mole (also called a dysplastic nevus). Although most dysplastic nevi do not develop into cancer, the chance is greater than with common moles, so they are almost always surgically removed. Dysplasia is usually caused by at least two genetic mutations—still not enough to cause cancer.

Carcinoma in situ is an even more advanced condition where the cells have all the cellular abnormalities of cancer under the microscope. Although it is sometimes called stage 0 cancer, it is not cancer because the abnormal cells do not invade nearby tissue the way cancer cells do. Because carcinomas in situ are even more likely to become cancer than dysplasia is, they are almost always treated with surgical removal.

Cancer biology: Facts and feelings

The core concepts in this chapter are essential for understanding how cancer comes to be. Hopefully, the bees and flower stories have helped explain the buzz about cancer stem cells. Before moving on I'd like to use my left brain and my right brain (figure 3.6) to summarize first the facts and then my feelings about what I have learned. My hope is

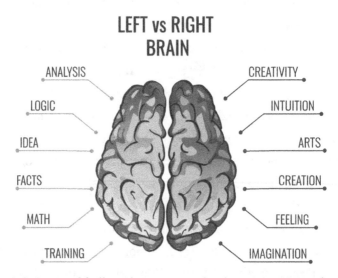

Figure 3.6. Facts and feelings about cancer. When it comes to cancer, the right brain often takes the lead.

that after finishing the book, the left brain, which is often dominated by the right when it comes to cancer, will eventually take charge.

The facts

1. Cancer is the consequence of mutations, or changes, that occur in genes involved in regulating and controlling normal cell growth and survival.

2. Mutations can be caused by environmental insults (such as cigarette smoking) or inherited from parents (such as *BRCA* mutations, which cause breast and ovarian cancer).

3. Most cancer-causing mutations appear to be random errors that develop as a natural consequence of the many normal cell divisions needed to keep us alive and healthy.

4. Cell division is extremely complicated and errors are expected, but most random errors or mutations are in parts of the DNA that have no effect on cell function. And the body's surveillance system, the immune system, is hard at work eliminating cells with mistakes.

5. Eventually, a mutation at a hotspot (a DNA segment that does affect cell function) will sneak past the surveillance system. But many sequential mutations are needed before cancer can progress. Most cancers are not detectable for many years and until billions of cancerous cells have replicated.

6. Cancer stem cells are organ stem cells that have mutated when replacing differentiated organ cells. They are long-lived cells, making it possible for the multiple mutations that are necessary for cancer progression to occur sequentially over time. Cancer stem cells also self-renew and thus allow the cancer to grow. Just like normal stem cells, which circulate in the bloodstream for organ repair, cancer stem cells can

circulate, or metastasize, even as early as the first cancer cell. This is why many treatments induce remission, but the disease may resurface.

7.   Despite what we all have been taught about cancer, it can never really be diagnosed early, as more than 85% of its life span has typically occurred by the time it is big enough to be diagnosed.

Now the feelings

In working on this chapter, I had mixed feelings. I learned that I could live a long time with cancer—and maybe even die with it—without even knowing. Strangely, this makes me feel good. Let me wax philosophical for a moment and pose a popular question: If a tree falls in the forest, does it make a sound? A simple definition of sound is a hearable noise or our perception of air vibrations. So a tree falling certainly disturbs the air and sends off air waves or vibrations, but arguably there is no sound if no one heard it. Bottom line: I don't care to know what crazy mutation party my cells might be having until I perceive it and I can possibly do something about it. Don't sign me up for a whole-body scan just yet.

I also learned that a cancer diagnosis is far from a death sentence. Some cancers won't shorten my life or even need to be treated. This also makes me feel good.

Finally, if cancer could be slowed or even stopped, it sure would be nice to know sooner rather than later. Researchers are tackling this very challenge by working on better diagnostic tests and earlier assessment of risk. I'm encouraged by this, and we will talk about it more.

CHAPTER 4

Metastasis

The Moving Target

WHEN MY MOM WAS DIAGNOSED WITH lung cancer, I asked Rick why surgery and radiation were not able to cure more patients with cancer. My family was thrilled to hear doctors say, "We got it early." Similarly, other patients and their families are equally elated when their surgeons say, "We got it all," but in the end that rarely seems to be the case. Radiation appeared to hold mom's lung cancer at bay for five years, at which time it progressed.

Surgery and radiation were the primary weapons in the battle against cancer for many years. Now those therapies are taking a back seat to chemotherapy, targeted therapies, and immunotherapy, especially as these new treatments become safer and more sophisticated. Patients rarely die from cancer at the initial site—surgery or radiation are often able to take care of that. Rather, they succumb to cancer that has spread, or metastasized, to distant sites.

When doctors say "we got it early," they mean that there are no signs the cancer has yet metastasized outside of the primary site, and thus radiation or surgery may be able to "get it all." As previously discussed, cancer is never diagnosed early; by the time of diagnosis, the majority of its life span has already transpired. Moreover, detecting metastases (mets) even as large as 100 million cells is extremely unlikely, making it virtually impossible to know that the cancer was found before it has spread. Thus, a surgeon can honestly say "I got all the cancer I could see" but can never know that surgery "got it all."

Since the metastatic spread, not the primary site of cancer, is usually what kills patients, is it possible that surgery, radiation, or any treatment will prevent mets? Rick tells me the answer is no, because the mutations responsible for mets, and thus the mets themselves, have likely already occurred by the time the cancer is diagnosed. Indeed, chemotherapy is now commonly applied after surgery or radiation treatment—so-called adjuvant therapy—in an often-failed attempt to eradicate the undetected mets while their cancer cell numbers are small. Since cancer mets are so critical to cancer outcomes, let's investigate why and how cancers spread in the first place.

Mets, cancer stem cells, and the microenvironment: Sowing the seeds of discontent

Most cancers start in adult organ stem cells that develop genetic mutations, causing them to grow abnormally. Normal stem cells can circulate for the purposes of tissue repair, like seeds in the wind. Just as seeds won't grow if the wind lands them in an inhospitable environment (like a road or sidewalk), normal organ stem cells lack the ability to grow outside the "soil" of their home organ microenvironment—a good thing, so that you don't grow a kidney in your liver or vice versa. This relationship between stem cells and their home environment is like swallows that migrate thousands of miles twice a year between North and South America but tend to return to the same nesting spots, where they feel at home. Similarly, when needed for tissue maintenance or repair, normal stem cells return home to the specialized microenvironment of their organs of origin, where they are best able to survive and grow.

In many ways, normal organ stem cells are more similar to each other than they are to their children, which make up the bulk of each organ. Another plant analogy will help illustrate this concept. It's easy to distinguish the blossom of a tulip from that of a daffodil or an iris. I bet that most of you, however, would be hard pressed to distinguish the roots of these flowers from one another, even with a picture (figure 4.1) because they look so similar. Even my wife, Ann, who spent a lot of time in our gardens, went to the local nursery, bought a bunch of bulbs, took them out of their labeled bags, and—since they only take on the characteristics of the plant once they start to grow—forgot which was which. Adult organ stem cells follow the same paradigm. Regardless of how different the organs look—breast, prostate, lung, kidney, thyroid—the stem cells look and behave similarly. They take on the characteristics of the organ only when they start to grow.

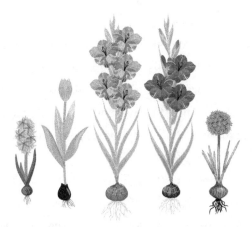

Figure 4.1. You may be able to recognize the flowers, but how about the roots? Similarly, it is difficult to recognize the organ of origin for normal stem cells and their cancerous counterparts.

Cancer stem cells are also more like the normal stem cells they arose from than they are like their children or progeny that form the bulk of the cancer. Like normal stem cells, they need a nurturing microenvironment to grow. Cancer stem cells obviously find their home microenvironment hospitable, or the cancer wouldn't have developed in the first place. In addition, random genetic mutations in cancer stem cells can confer these abnormal descendants of normal organ stem cells with the ability to grow outside of their normal microenvironment and thus metastasize to other sites. Let's now consider several different cancers that illustrate specific aspects of how the interaction of cancer stem cells and the microenvironment influences metastatic growth.

Blood cancers: Born to run

The job of white blood cells is to circulate through the body looking for infections, so it is not surprising that the cancers that develop from these cells also move around the blood. Despite being "born to run" in the blood system, blood cancers rarely grow, or become metastatic, outside that system. Rather, blood cancers tend to remain "at home" in their nurturing microenvironments with their normal counterparts. Multiple myeloma cells thrive in the bone marrow with the normal noncancerous plasma cells, the cells that make antibodies to fight infections. Leukemia stays with normal white blood cells in the blood and bone marrow. And lymphomas enjoy the comfort of lymph nodes with normal lymphocytes.

Lymphomas were once thought to circulate less than leukemias. Surgery was never a major component in the treatment of lymphomas (think of trying to use a knife to cut blood); the treatment of choice was radiation. The Ann Arbor staging system was developed to determine who could be cured with radiation. Stage I or II (localized or early stage) was felt to be curable with radiation, while stage III or IV (advanced stage) required chemotherapy.

We now know that lymphomas are almost never localized—unsurprising since their normal counterparts, lymphocytes, continually circulate like other blood cells. Thus radiation is not curative for most lymphomas, although it can be used palliatively or to reduce symptoms from localized lymphoma masses. Although lymphomas usually remain in lymph nodes, by the time of diagnosis they are almost always in all lymph nodes in the body, often below the level of detection. Lymph nodes, which number in the hundreds throughout the body (figure 4.2), are the nests where lymphocytes develop and like to live. Tonsils are lymph nodes, and the spleen could be considered the biggest lymph node in the body.

Hodgkin lymphoma was once considered to be the quintessential cancer that could be cured with radiation. For decades, doctors believed Hodgkin lymphoma remained localized in one lymph node area until late in the disease and then moved to nearby lymph nodes through the lymphatic system (figure 4.2). Rick's laboratory showed, however, that Hodgkin lymphoma cells can be found in the blood of nearly every patient with Hodgkin lymphoma, even those with the disease at an early stage, when it is supposedly localized. Therefore, the treatment paradigm for Hodgkin lymphoma now includes chemotherapy, as it does for other types of lymphomas (often called non-Hodgkin lymphomas).

Brain cancer: The last to leave

The ability of cancers to metastasize should now seem obvious, since cancer stem cells arise from normal stem cells that circulate in the blood for the purpose of maintenance and repair of organs. And without question, the cause of most solid organ (lung, colon, breast,

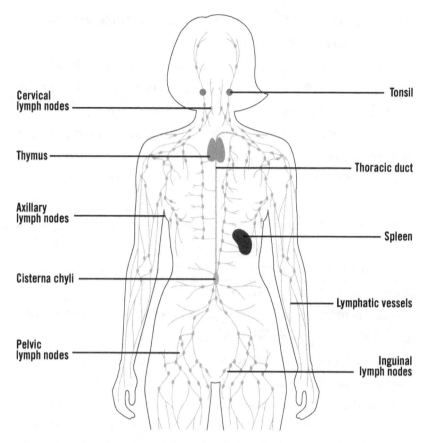

Figure 4.2. Lymph nodes and the rest of the lymphatic system, where lymphocytes live and travel when not in the bloodstream.

prostate, and so on) cancer deaths is the mets. An interesting exception is brain cancer. Although most brain cancers are highly aggressive, incurable, and usually fatal within a few years, clinically significant mets outside the brain are uncommon. This fact has led many oncologists to believe that brain cancer cells rarely if ever leave the brain. In fact, mets outside the brain were thought to be so rare that patients with brain cancer were allowed to donate organs after death. Surgery and radiation have been the mainstays of brain cancer treatment, but unfortunately these treatments are never curative.

The most common form of brain cancer is called glioblastoma multiforme (GBM for short). Surgery and radiation are unable to cure GBM because the cancer spreads locally, often to multiple non-adjacent areas in the brain. While GBM cells from the primary lesions could reach adjacent areas by "crawling" through tight spaces, they can spread to the other side of the brain only through the blood. Rick's laboratory has been able to find brain cancer cells circulating in the blood in many GBM patients, even at initial diagnosis. Moreover, several people who received donated organs from patients with GBM have developed cancer in their transplanted organs.

Notwithstanding the heading of this section, brain cancer is not really the last cancer to leave its primary site; as with other cancers, GBM cells circulate early in the disease. The mets don't show up because, like Hodgkin lymphoma cells (which were similarly thought at one point not to leave their initial lymph node site) and migrating swallows, GBM cells often do not find a suitable nest to migrate to outside the brain. Even when they do, most patients with GBM die from the disease in their brains before their mets are large enough to be detected.

BLT with a kosher pickle: There's no place like bone

Because bone marrow is the home of blood cells, all blood cancers—not just leukemias but also lymphomas and multiple myeloma—are often found in the bone marrow. Perhaps surprisingly, bone is also the most frequent site of mets in certain other cancers. "BLT with a kosher pickle" is the mnemonic taught in medical school to help students remember those cancers that commonly metastasize to bone: Breast, Lung, Thyroid, Kidney, and Prostate (figure 4.3).

When non-blood-cancer stem cells reach the bone marrow, they find it a hospitable microenvironment. Normal blood stem cells need

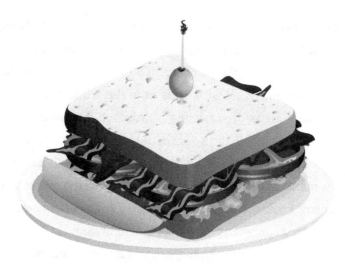

Figure 4.3. BLT with a Kosher Pickle. Even after Rick became a (mostly) vegetarian, this remains his favorite deli offering since he considers bacon just a condiment for the bread and vegetables. As an added benefit, it is also the mnemonic Rick was taught in medical school for remembering the cancers that commonly metastasize to bone: Breast, Lung, Thyroid, Kidney, and Prostate.

a special home that allows them to make new blood cells. This home needs to protect blood stem cells from the elements, as well as nurture and care for them. That is why the marrow is surrounded by a protective metal case (yes, the calcium that makes our bones and teeth strong is actually a metal) and has a complex microenvironment that also protects stem cells by inactivating toxins. The bone marrow also supplies special external signals to maintain normal blood stem cells and foster their growth. Cancer stem cells can benefit from these signals as well. Thus, as cancer stem cells circulate and pass through the bone marrow, instead of continuing their journey through the bloodstream, they often take a rest in the marrow, a sort of five-star hotel for stem cells.

It's not unheard of for breast cancer that appeared localized and was treated with curative intent to show up in bone 10–15 years later.

One of the main functions of the bone marrow microenvironment is to give normal blood stem cells a place to rest (or be dormant). Much of the life cycle of normal stem cells, like that of humans and animals, is spent in dormancy. Similar to sleep, this dormancy is a restorative period for the stem cells. In times of limited stress to an organ like the bone marrow, normal stem cells may divide only occasionally, essentially hibernating, sometimes for decades, until they are needed to replenish the organ (think Rip Van Winkle). The bone marrow microenvironment is fine-tuned to keep the stem cells happy while they hibernate.

Based on work conducted in Rick's laboratory and many others, we are just beginning to understand the highly regulated processes that control when normal stem cells are dormant and when they divide. Some data suggest that even normal organ adult stem cells may visit the bone marrow and rest. The bone marrow allows cancer stem cells to rest using the same processes it uses with normal stem cells. Surprisingly, this period of dormancy may occur even while cancer is growing fast in its site of origin. Why do stem cells rest, and what triggers a dormant cancer stem cell to awaken like good old Rip Van Winkle?

Both doctors and patients have wondered whether physical or emotional stress to an individual could trigger an awakening of cancer stem cells, particularly those resting in the bone marrow. For example, hormones that go up during pregnancy can be growth factors for breast cancer and other cancers. However, the National Cancer Institute has concluded that there is currently no strong clinical evidence that stress can lead to cancer recurrence. More likely, as we already discussed, a dormant cancer is awakened by an additional mutation that renders cancer stem cells no longer sensitive to the microenvironmental signals that triggered dormancy in the marrow.

Nevertheless, the interplay of stress and cancer remains an area of active research, and stress can certainly make dealing with cancer more difficult for both patients and caregivers.

Although the bone marrow is one of the most common sites, mets can occur in essentially any organ. Both normal and cancer stem cells are made to circulate. When they leave home and where they end up are based on two factors: how hospitable they find the organ and how "accomplished" they have become. The bone marrow, as noted, is hospitable to most stem cells, normal and cancer. Other hospitable sites are the liver and the lungs, two of the most common sites of mets other than bone and lymph nodes. The liver has a microenvironment similar to bone marrow, and in fact that is where blood stem cells are born in the fetus. In addition, the blood supply from all the gastrointestinal organs runs through the liver, which removes toxins that may have been ingested, before going to the rest of the body. The lungs are highly oxygenated, a feature that most cells, including cancer cells, find welcoming.

The other major determinant of metastatic ability is how "accomplished" the cancer has become. Cancer stem cells that have developed lots of mutations are often able to bring their microenvironment with them or even transform the foreign microenvironment to suit their needs, a little like the early pioneers making their homes out in the wilderness.

It is not unusual for mets to be found before the primary cancer site. Rick diagnosed his mom's pancreatic cancer at her 70th birthday party when she told him about pain in the right side of her belly that she had been having for over a month. She was not particularly concerned, thinking it was probably a pulled muscle, except that it wasn't getting better. In fact, it was the mets in her liver that were giving her pain and where the disease was seen on scans. The primary lesion in her pancreas was small and hard to see. The liver appeared to provide an even more hospitable environment for the cancer cells than their primary home, the pancreas. Most consider pancreatic cancer, like my mom's lung cancer, especially when metastatic, an immediate death sentence. Rick's mom, however, entered a complete remission with chemotherapy and lived and enjoyed her grandchildren for two more years.

Attacking mets: Hitting the moving target

Since surgery or radiation can generally deal with the local effects of cancer, the real enemy is not the original site of the cancer, but the mets. Not only are they destructive, but they are likely to pop up in multiple places, even if they are not yet detectable. They are also difficult to treat, not only because cancer stem cells maintain normal stem cell hardiness but also because their microenvironment itself inactivates toxins, including chemotherapy.

Don't worry! There are silver linings in these dark clouds. Mets have two characteristics that can make them easier to target with therapies. The number of cells in mets, particularly before they are detectable, is small—usually orders of magnitude less than the initial cancer site at diagnosis. The cells making up mets are also often less heterogeneous.

Since most cancers are metastatic at diagnosis, doesn't it make sense to treat the mets before they are detectable? This is exactly the concept behind adjuvant therapy. For example, after surgery to remove the visible evidence of breast cancer, adjuvant chemotherapy is given to attack the present but undetectable mets. Adjuvant therapy is also called maintenance therapy (it is meant to maintain a remission). We'll talk more about attacking mets later.

Summary: Should I stay or should I go?

Since cancer stem cells can circulate in the blood from day one, let's summarize the biology of mets by answering the question posed by the rock group the Clash: "Should I stay or should I go?" (one of *Rolling Stone*'s 500 Greatest Songs of All Time). When do cancer stem cells stay or go; that is, if, when, and where do cancer stem cells metastasize?

Step 1. An organ stem cell mutates, creating a cancer stem cell.

Step 2. Like their normal counterparts, whose job is organ repair, cancer stem cells have the capacity to leave their "home" organ and circulate throughout the body.

Step 3. Despite the ability to migrate, cancer stem cells often end up back at their original home (like a swallow or your child after college), because there really is no place like home.

Step 4. When the cancer stem cell leaves "home," it finds a hospitable foreign microenvironment like the bone marrow, liver, or lung.

Step 5. The new organ system is so hospitable that the cancer stem cell often decides to rest (or become dormant). This dormancy is what leads to late relapses following long remissions, as sometimes seen in breast cancer and other cancers.

Step 6. Through additional mutations, the cancer stem cells eventually become independent enough to make their own microenvironment in the new organ system, creating a detectable met.

CHAPTER 5

Clinical Basics

Bench to Bedside and Back Again

FOR RICK, THE MOST GRATIFYING experience as a cancer doctor is making a discovery in the laboratory (the bench) and turning it into something that helps the patient clinically (the bedside). Such bench-to-bedside research is called translational research. Much of what has been learned about cancer comes from research that goes the other way as well: clues from the bedside influence work that is done at the laboratory bench (figure 5.1). Although the last couple of chapters focused on biology (the bench), the rest of the book will concentrate mostly on clinical aspects of cancer (the bedside). When treating patients, Rick spends a good deal of time explaining the biology of their cancer to help them better understand how the disease behaves clinically. Let's take what we learned from the bench in the last three chapters and see how it helps us understand the basics of cancer at the bedside.

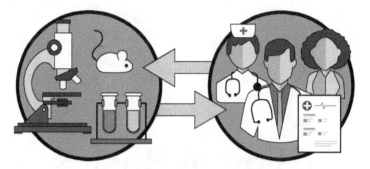

Figure 5.1. Bench to bedside and back. Cancer research is bidirectional: laboratory discoveries lead to clinical improvements, and clinical observations influence further laboratory research.

Cancer types: What's in a name?

It used to be said that there were about 100 different types of cancer. Cancers were named according to the organs where they started: lung cancer or breast cancer or colon cancer. Some types of organ cancers were further classified by their appearance under the microscope, such as small cell cancer of the lung. Nowadays, naming cancers for their organ of origin is no longer sufficient to define the cancer. Saying a patient has lung cancer or breast cancer is no different from saying they have cancer, since so many different types of cancers can arise from any organ. We now know that there are thousands, perhaps even tens of thousands, of different cancers.

Cancers are now best defined by the genetic mutations that cause the cancer. It is these mutations, not the organ it arises from or how it appears under the microscope, that determine the behavior of a cancer. For the purposes of understanding cancer and its treatment, how cancers grow and behave may be a better way of classifying them than the organs they arise from.

Cancers are further classified using several different staging systems. Broadly, a cancer's stage refers to its extent at diagnosis,

SCIENCE CORNER

Cancer Staging Systems

The TNM Classification of Malignant Tumors is the most commonly used system for classifying the stages of cancer.

- *T* describes the size of the original (primary) tumor and whether it has invaded nearby tissue.
- *N* describes nearby (regional) lymph nodes that are involved.
- *M* describes distant metastasis (the spread of cancer from one part of the body to another).

In the TNM system, numbers after each letter give more details about the cancer—for example, T1N0MX or T3N1M0. Here's what the letters and numbers mean:

- Primary tumor (T)
  - TX: The main tumor cannot be measured.
  - T0: The main tumor cannot be found.
  - T1, T2, T3, T4: The numbers refer to the size and/or extent of the main tumor. The higher the number after the T, the larger the tumor or the more it has grown into nearby tissues.
- Regional lymph nodes (N)
  - NX: Cancer in nearby lymph nodes cannot be measured.
  - N0: There is no cancer in nearby lymph nodes.
  - N1, N2, N3: The numbers refer to the number and location of lymph nodes that contain cancer. The higher the number after the N, the more lymph nodes contain cancer.
- Distant metastasis (M)
  - MX: Metastasis cannot be measured.
  - M0: Cancer has not spread to other parts of the body.
  - M1: Cancer has spread to other parts of the body.

For some cancers, the staging is grouped into five less-detailed stages. Lymphomas, discussed in the next Science Corner, use this system. The stages in this system are as follows:

- *Stage 0* describes cancer in situ.
- *Stage I* is usually a small cancer that has not grown deeply into nearby tissues or spread to the lymph nodes or other parts of the body. It is often called early-stage cancer.
- *Stage II* and *Stage III* indicate larger cancers or tumors that have grown more deeply into nearby tissue. They may also have spread to lymph nodes but not to other parts of the body.
- *Stage IV* means that the cancer has spread to other organs or parts of the body. It may also be called advanced or metastatic cancer.

especially how large it is and the magnitude of its spread. These staging systems were initially developed to help determine the prognosis of cancers and which ones would benefit from surgery, radiation, or both.

As treatments for cancer improve, classical staging systems become less useful. Not only do new, more effective therapies change the prognostic implications of staging systems but also, as will be discussed in chapter 8 ("Cancer Treatments"), surgery and radiation are being used less often. Staging now plays little role in blood cancers such as leukemias because the cancerous blood cells in these diseases are always spread throughout the body at diagnosis, even if they appear localized. Moreover, treatments for blood cancers have improved, so many staging characteristics that used to predict outcomes no longer do.

When talking to patients, Rick relies on a simpler classification system that is both easy to understand and highly relevant to current thinking about prognosis and therapies. The thousands of different cancer types, he says, can all be lumped into three main categories:

- fast-growing cancers that are curable
- slow-growing or indolent cancers that are relatively well behaved
- aggressive cancers that are incurable

Perhaps because Rick deals exclusively with blood cancers, he tells me it is possible to understand essentially everything about cancer from one broad category of blood cancers called lymphomas. Lymphomas are cancers arising from lymphocytes (usually B lymphocytes), which are the blood cells responsible for fighting infections by traveling around the body. Lymphomas are the most common form of blood cancers, and their genetics and biology are among the best understood (see the Science Corner on the genetics of lymphomas). Like cancer in general, lymphomas come in many different varieties but can largely be grouped into the three broad categories above.

Fast-growing cancers that are curable: Overpopulating by having lots of babies

Fast-growing cancers that are curable represent what some of us think of as cancer but actually encompass only a small percentage of cases. The story of this type of lymphoma starts with the Irish surgeon Denis Burkitt. Burkitt entered Trinity College in Dublin, Ireland, in 1929 to study engineering but transferred to medicine, passing the Royal College of Surgeons examination in 1938. During World War II Burkitt served with the Royal Army Medical Corps in Africa, and after the war he decided his calling lay in helping the people of Uganda, both medically and spiritually.

In 1958 he published a description of an unusual tumor that would often show up on the jaws of children in Uganda but could also occur in other areas of the body. These tumors grew rapidly—doubling every 12 to 24 hours—and the affected children would usually die in a matter of days or weeks. Working with pathologists in Uganda, Burkitt demonstrated that the tumor consisted of cancerous lymphocytes. Radiation therapy was not available in tropical Africa, and the cancer's rapid growth in widespread sites precluded any hope of success with surgery, so Burkitt began treating these children with chemotherapy trials. He collected supplies of chemotherapy agents, particularly cyclophosphamide, which had just been approved in the late 1950s, and used them unconventionally, in relatively small doses, because of the absence of sophisticated facilities to care for cancer patients. He found that relatively low doses of single chemotherapy drugs were able to produce astonishing regressions and occasionally even cures.

Although we now use multiagent chemotherapy regimens and cure most patients with the lymphoma that now bears Burkitt's name, these responses to a single drug highlight how sensitive Burkitt lymphoma is to chemotherapy despite being widespread at diagnosis. Like lymphocytes, which move around the body looking for infections, lymphoma cells travel around the body, so even though the mets in Burkitt lymphoma may be too small to be detected at first, the disease is almost always widespread, or metastatic, at diagnosis.

So why is this specific cancer so curable? I'll give you the quick answer. Chemotherapy is highly effective at killing cells that divide rapidly, and Burkitt lymphoma is perhaps the fastest-growing human cancer. In addition to Burkitt lymphoma, several other fast-growing lymphomas, such as Hodgkin lymphoma and diffuse large B-cell lymphoma, can be cured with chemotherapy. Some leukemias (but certainly not all) and testicular lymphoma also fall into this fast-growing, curable category of cancers.

SCIENCE CORNER

Genetics of Lymphomas

The machinery for the work of each and every cell in the body is contained within the 46 chromosomes present in all cells but is turned off in cells where it isn't needed. Since the job of B lymphocytes is to make antibodies, the machinery to do this is always turned on in these cells.

To make antibodies that can recognize an unlimited number of unique and diverse antigens, B lymphocytes must rearrange their genes involved in this process. This rearranging of segments of the antibody genes is what permits the cells to manufacture so many different antibodies. Just as the complicated process of copying DNA during cell division does not always happen perfectly, so too this complicated process of rearranging antibody genes can go wrong.

During one of these mistakes in this process, the main antibody gene, which is located on chromosome 14 and is switched on in B lymphocytes, may by chance move next to a gene involved in cell growth. This growth gene, which is meant to function only during the process of making new cells (cell division), gets switched on as a consequence of being next to, and under the influence of, the antibody gene. This type of mistake happens in most lymphomas, and the type of lymphoma that develops depends on which growth gene mistakenly moves next to the antibody gene on chromosome 14 and becomes active.

In Burkitt lymphoma, perhaps the most important gene involved in cell division, MYC on chromosome 8, is moved next to the antibody gene on chromosome 14 (translocation 8;14) so that MYC is always on. Having MYC always on is like putting a brick on the gas pedal of cell division, causing the cells to divide very fast. Indeed, Burkitt lymphoma cells divide so fast that they use up their energy supplies and begin to die on their own. Chemotherapy is able to push these already dying cells over the edge—this is the genesis of the well-known concept that chemotherapy kills cells that are dividing fast.

Now what happens if a different gene—say, one involved in promoting the survival of a cell—gets moved next to the antibody gene on chromosome 14 during the process of antibody gene rearrangement in B lymphocytes? The cell will be expected to live longer than it should. This is exactly what happens in follicular lymphoma, one of the commonest lymphomas. In this case, the gene moving next to the antibody gene on chromosome 14 is BCL-2 on chromosome 18, one of the most important genes that keep cells alive by preventing the process of cell death or apoptosis. The translocation (14;18) makes too much Bcl-2, causing lymphoma cells not only to live too long but also to fail to die even after chemotherapy, making this form of lymphoma generally incurable with standard therapies, although it can be well behaved for decades.

Slow-growing, well-behaved cancers that live too long can develop additional genetic mutations and become more aggressive in a process called transformation. The classic transformation event in follicular lymphoma involves the same mutation seen in Burkitt lymphoma, so that MYC is now turned on, converting what was previously an indolent, long-lived lymphoma because of too much Bcl-2 into one that is also fast growing.

If you stopped off in the Science Corner on the genetics of lymphomas, you may have found it a bit hard to follow with all the DNA copying and antibody segment rearranging. Just think about how difficult it was to figure this all out in the first place. We included this and similar examples to help you appreciate the incredible progress that is being made in understanding and treating cancer through DNA mapping. We are fortunate to have generations of gifted scientists who have contributed and continue to contribute to cancer research.

Let's return briefly to Denis Burkitt. Since the childhood form of the lymphoma that bears his name was endemic to the malaria belt in equatorial Africa, he hypothesized that the lymphoma might be caused by an infection. His colleagues eventually showed that the virus that causes mononucleosis, the Epstein-Barr virus (EBV), was present in essentially all the lymphoma cells. This finding initially led many cancer researchers to believe that viruses were important in the development of all cancer, though it turns out that viral-induced cancer is relatively uncommon. Even the role of EBV in Burkitt lymphoma remains unclear; although all Burkitt lymphomas are caused by the translocation of chromosomes 8 and 14, EBV is not present in most cases of Burkitt lymphoma outside of Africa.

Slow-growing or indolent cancers: Overpopulating by living longer

Instead of speeding along with the pedal to the metal, some cancer cells are programmed to not die, just like car trips that seem like they will never end. What happens if the genetic mutation causes the cancer to live too long instead of grow too fast? This is exactly what happens in follicular lymphoma, one of the commonest lymphomas. Even chemotherapy doesn't kill follicular lymphoma cells, making the disease generally incurable with standard therapies.

Follicular lymphoma cancer cells actually tend to grow even more slowly than their normal counterparts. Accordingly, patients with this type of lymphoma actually have a median survival period of about 20 years. Early treatment of this disease, before the patient is bothered by the lymphoma, does not change the prognosis, because the lymphoma is incurable. I suspect many would consider a diagnosis of lymphoma a death sentence, so it might come as a surprise that people with one of the most common forms of lymphoma can survive so long in the absence of a cure. Since the median age of onset of follicular lymphoma is between 65 and 70, many patients will die with the lymphoma rather than from it. Moreover, DNA damage from chemotherapy or radiation can produce additional mutations that cause the lymphoma to change behavior (see next section below). Accordingly, many patients with follicular lymphoma are just observed rather than treated. Other cancers caused by gene mutations that lead cancer cells to live too long include chronic lymphocytic leukemia, chronic myeloid leukemia, some forms of multiple myeloma and myelodysplastic syndromes (MDSs), and prostate cancer.

Aggressive cancers that are incurable: Lots of babies and lots of old folks

Our final and the most common type of cancer is like the never-ending car trip with someone who starts out driving well but then turns into a maniac. Initially, these cancers are usually caused by a mutation that causes them to live too long, and as such they are typically also slow growing and incurable. Most indolent cancers, however, have another important characteristic: they can change behavior and become aggressive. The genetic mutation that prevents them from undergoing apoptosis—that is, dying—also sets the stage for additional DNA mutations that could arise from chemotherapy or radiation. In addition, these cancers may develop further genetic damage from mistakes during normal cell division.

Yes, chemotherapy that isn't curative can actually make cancer worse. Cells have a process to repair DNA, but this process is successful only if the DNA damage is not extensive. A cell will try to repair even extensive damage to the two complementary DNA strands by randomly adding base pairs to fill in the damaged strands. It's no surprise that with no DNA guide or template to follow, the repair can produce mistakes or mutations. Normally, cells can sense such extensive damage and activate the apoptotic pathway of orderly cell suicide to clean up the mess. However, if the apoptotic pathway is blocked by too much Bcl-2 or other cell survival cancer gene mutations like *BCR-ABL* or the Philadelphia chromosome (a translocation of two normal genes that should not be next to one another in chronic myeloid leukemia), the cell's attempt to repair the DNA without a template will proceed, resulting in additional mutations. If one of these mutations leads to faster cell division, now you have a cancer that not only can't be killed (from a block in the apoptosis pathway) but also grows too fast.

This process, in which slow-growing, well-behaved cancers become more aggressive through additional mutations, is called transformation. The classic transformation event in follicular lymphoma occurs when the cancer acquires the same mutation seen in Burkitt lymphoma, so that it both becomes incurable with standard therapy and grows fast.

Most solid-organ cancers like lung and colon cancer develop in a similar manner, which makes them so difficult to treat. Like follicular lymphoma, these solid-organ cancers usually start out with anti-apoptotic mutations, which makes them long lived and incurable but also well behaved for a while (colon polyps are an example). They then acquire the additional mutations that make the cells divide too fast, resulting in fast-growing, incurable cancers.

Cancer and KISS

KISS here does not refer to anything French, one of my favorite candies, or dudes wanting to "rock and roll all night and party every day" (figure 5.2). Rather, it signifies "Keep it simple, stupid." Cancer is complicated. You can see from the discussion of specific genetic mutations in the examples given (such as *BCL-2* and *MYC*) the extent to which cancer is studied, understood, and sometimes treated at this level. If you have had a detailed discussion with an oncologist about a cancer diagnosis—your own, a family member's, or a friend's—then you have likely had to try to understand a flood of genetic information that is often the basis for identifying a specific cancer and treating

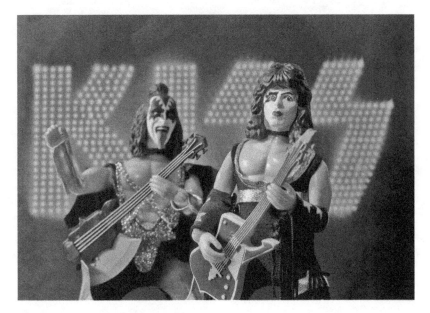

Figure 5.2. Keep it simple, stupid.

it. Now we hope you are better prepared to ask some simple, yet critical, questions:

- What type of cancer is it and where did it start?
- Is that specific cancer
  - a fast-growing cancer and curable?
  - a slow-growing or indolent cancer that is relatively well behaved?
  - an aggressive cancer that is incurable?
- Is there any indication that the cancer has spread to nearby tissue or to other organs?

CHAPTER 6

Treatment versus Cure

Of Flies, Flyswatters, Dandelions, and Lawn Mowers

OVER THE PAST TWO DECADES, the Food and Drug Administration (FDA) has approved more than 100 new anticancer treatments. It's an impressive track record, especially when compared with new anticancer treatment approvals over the past century: less than 10 approvals before 1960 and only 27 by 1975. In 2018 and 2019 alone, the FDA approved 30 new anticancer treatments. The increased pace of new anticancer drug approvals has led to improved survival for many patients with cancer and even some cures. Approval required all of these drugs to show some clinical benefit, as documented by objective measurements of cancer response, improvements in quality of life as assessed by questionnaires, or a delay in recurrence. And of course, the negative side effects of these drugs had to be known and acceptable.

Clinical response: How much is enough?

The clinical development of new anticancer treatments—clinical trials—usually proceeds through sequential steps called phases (figure 6.1). In general, clinical trials are designed to identify (1) safe treatment doses and frequencies, (2) any negative side effects on the body, and (3) of course, cancer-fighting benefits.

- Phase 1 trials, usually involving small numbers of patients, establish safe drug doses and look for the first hints of clinical activity, such as a reduction in the size of the cancerous mass.
- Phase 2 trials, usually including hundreds of people, focus on the effects of new therapies in treating specific cancers.
- Phase 3 trials often involve hundreds to thousands of patients in order to compare the effectiveness of new treatments with current standard therapies.
- Less common are very early (phase 0) and later (phase 4) clinical trials. Phase 0 trials are extremely small trials that help researchers decide whether a new agent should be tested in phase 1 trials. Phase 4 trials take place after a new treatment has been approved and is on the market to assess long-term safety and effectiveness.

Clinical Trials

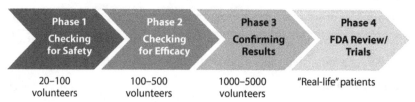

Phase 1 — Checking for Safety — 20–100 volunteers

Phase 2 — Checking for Efficacy — 100–500 volunteers

Phase 3 — Confirming Results — 1000–5000 volunteers

Phase 4 — FDA Review/Trials — "Real-life" patients

Figure 6.1. Clinical trial phases. The clinical trial development of new anticancer treatments usually proceeds through sequential steps called phases.

- Most new therapies will ultimately not be used alone, and further development of combination strategies likewise requires sequential steps.

The success of new anticancer agents in these trials is usually defined by their ability to produce a clinical response—in other words, to shrink the cancer. A partial response (also called a partial remission) means that the size of the cancer has gone down by at least half, as measured by standard two-dimensional x-rays. To achieve a partial remission, a cancer mass measuring 10 centimeters in one direction by 10 cm in the other (or 100 cm²) would have to shrink to 7 cm by 7 cm, or 49 cm². Although the standard definition of partial remission relies on two-dimensional measurements, a cancer mass has three dimensions, and our example actually represents more than a 50% reduction in volume using three-dimensional measurements: $7 \times 7 \times 7$ (or 343 cm³) is a reduction of two-thirds from $10 \times 10 \times 10$ (or 1,000 cm³). A complete response (also called a complete remission) means that all detectable evidence of the cancer has vanished. Any result less than a partial remission is considered to be no response. New anticancer agents that can induce partial remissions are usually deemed successes, and the ability to produce a complete remission is heralded as a major advance.

A cardinal principle of treating cancer has been that a clinical response (a measurable reduction in the cancer) will translate into a clinical benefit (a reduction in symptoms and especially improved survival) without significant irreversible effects on quality of life. Moreover, the major advantage of using clinical response as a primary trial end point is that it is measurable over weeks to months, allowing the stepwise process of drug development to occur rapidly and efficiently. In contrast, demonstrating a delay in the time to recurrence or an improvement in overall survival or, even better, cure (the disease never comes back) adds significant complexity to trial design, usually requiring trials with large patient numbers and long follow-up.

If the size or location of the cancer is causing symptoms, a measurable response clearly can produce a clinical benefit by decreasing side effects caused by the cancer and improving quality of life. It is often the case, however, that clinical responses do not translate into cures or even improved survival. In fact, there are numerous well-accepted examples where response and survival do not correlate. Indolent lymphoma patients who achieve complete remissions do not experience survival advantages over similar patients treated with a "watch and wait" approach. Similarly, responses have not usually translated into survival benefits in prostate cancer. Further, despite many new treatments for metastatic breast cancer, survival has been minimally impacted. Even when responses are associated with statistically significant improvements in survival, the survival advantage is often incrementally small, frequently a few weeks to months.

In actuality, the major rationale for the use of measurable clinical response as a surrogate for effectiveness of therapy is the premise that a complete remission must precede cure. Since cure can currently be established only through long-term follow-up, a complete remission will always precede verification of cure. Surprisingly, however, a complete remission by standard criteria may be neither a prerequisite nor a requirement for disease control and prolonged survival. Let's dive into the apparent paradox that treatment response and survival in cancer are not necessarily linked.

The kinetics of cancer cell kill: Flies and flyswatters

The biggest claims to fame of our alma mater, Bucknell, are alumni Hall of Fame pitcher Christy Mathewson and Pulitzer Prize-winning author Philip Roth. But this small liberal arts institution in rural central Pennsylvania also spawned an unusual number of accomplished cancer researchers. At the start of this millennium, research on hematologic malignancies (blood cancers) at three of the best-known cancer hospitals (Johns Hopkins, Massachusetts General, and Moffitt) was led by people who had graduated within a year of each other from Bucknell (Rick, plus two other alumni).

While I was switching majors from math to religion, Rick was persevering in his major, chemistry. When we started this book, he made me promise that I would let him bring in one basic principle from that important scientific discipline. I agreed, thinking that I would be able to understand *one* chemistry principle. So here is my one basic idea from chemistry: the principle of first-order kinetics, which helps explain how cancers respond to chemotherapy.

As applied to cancer treatment, first-order kinetics means that a specific dose of chemotherapy will kill a constant fraction of the cancer cells that are present in a patient rather than a constant number of cancer cells. This is one of the many reasons that partial remissions (which shrink cancers by 50% or more) often do not translate into improved overall survival. Rick uses the analogy of swatting flies while blindfolded to explain first-order kinetics to his patients, to help them understand why a chemotherapy drug often is less effective than it may appear (see the Science Corner on first-order kinetics).

Cancer heterogeneity: Flies, super flies, and lord of the flies

What happens if one in a trillion flies (or cancer cells) is born with a random genetic mutation that provides it with exceptional flying speed, allowing it to avoid the flyswatter better than other flies? Perhaps another is born with extraordinary vision that also helps it avoid the flyswatter. These two flies could mate and have fast-flying, keen-eyed super flies (figure 6.2) that an aimless swat will never get. You are probably thinking, take off the blindfold—use better, more targeted chemotherapy—but we know how hard it can be to swat a fast-flying insect even when it can be seen. Random genetic mutations that occur as one cancer cell multiplies to become the trillion cells

SCIENCE CORNER

Chemotherapy and First-Order Kinetics

First-order kinetics, when applied to cancer chemotherapy, means that the dose of the chemotherapy drug will kill the same fraction, not the same number, of cancer cells in successive rounds. To illustrate, let's consider a room full of flies and a blindfolded person with a flyswatter aimlessly wandering around the room swatting at the flies at a constant rate. In this analogy, the flies represent the cancer cells and the flyswatter the chemotherapy. Let's say the room initially held 100 million flies. At the end of an hour of swatting (which represents a round of chemotherapy), the flies are counted, and 10 million flies remain. Thus, the flyswatter killed 90% of the flies.

So, using first-order kinetics, how many of the remaining 10 million flies will the blindfolded individual kill during a second hour of fly swatting (representing a second round of chemotherapy)? Certainly not 90 million again, since only 10 million are left. This time around, our aimless flyswatter will hit the same amount of air—90%—again killing 90% of the flies, or 9 million (90% of 10 million), leaving 1 million flies in the room. So what happens when there are only 10 flies in the room? Yep, 90% of the air will be swatted, and one fly will survive.

We all know that flies are smarter and faster than this example would allow (we'll get into this in a bit), but the concept and underlying math are powerful tools for understanding chemotherapy outcomes. As with the flyswatter, the same dose of chemotherapy would be expected to kill the same fraction, not the same number, of cancer cells. When a cancer is diagnosed, there are at least 100 billion (11 logs), and usually a trillion, cancer cells present. It takes the same dose of chemotherapy to kill the first 90% of cancer cells (90% of 1 trillion is 900 billion) as it does to kill the last 90% (9 of the last 10 cells).

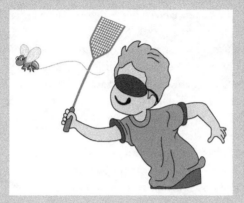

This youngster clearly enjoys learning first-order kinetics.

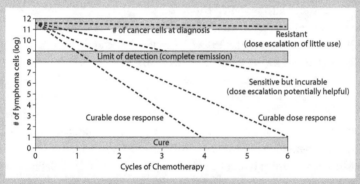

Graphical representation of how effective the same dose of chemotherapy is against different cancers. The steeper the slope of the line, the more sensitive the cancer is to chemotherapy. The flatter the line, the more resistant the cancer is to chemotherapy.

The graph shows dose-response lines—visual representations of how effective the same dose of chemotherapy is against four different cancers. The steeper the slope of the line, the more sensitive the cancer is to chemotherapy. The flatter the line, the more resistant the cancer is to chemotherapy. The two steepest lines (labeled "curable dose responses") represent two cancers that can be cured with six cycles of chemotherapy. The graph makes it apparent that for a cancer to be

(*continued*)

cured with six cycles of chemotherapy, you have to kill at least two logs (99%) of cancer cells with each dose. With that dose response, the cancer will consist of fewer than 100 million (10^8 or 8 logs) cells after just two cycles and hence no longer be detectable (or in complete remission).

Some leukemias, fast-growing lymphomas, and testicular cancers are essentially the only cancers that display such steep dose-response slopes to standard chemotherapy and are hence curable. The figure's top line ("resistant"), with a flat slope, depicts the response to chemotherapy exhibited by most solid tumors. Cancer doctors feel fortunate when they see a partial remission (that is, a reduction in size by two-thirds), but as the top line shows, killing less than 1 log (90%) of cancer cells accomplishes little in the battle to cure the cancer. In such cancers it would also be futile to increase the numbers of cycles or the dose of chemotherapy (a larger flyswatter), since it would be virtually impossible to ever achieve a dose that can kill 12 logs.

The second line from the top ("sensitive but incurable") represents the situation where standard dose chemotherapy is able to reduce the number of cancer cells below the limit of detection (a complete remission, or fewer than 100 million cells). It may be possible to cure such cancers—which include some leukemias, some fast-growing lymphomas, and testicular cancers—by increasing the dosage.

Curing a cancer, as represented by the bottom two dose-response lines, assumes that all the cells in the cancer show similar responsiveness to chemotherapy. However, we know that this is not true of most cancers because of tumor heterogeneity. Moreover, even if all the cells within a cancer are initially sensitive to chemotherapy, new cancer cells are continually being made (flies are missed by the swatter or, while the flyswatter rests, continue to breed), further increasing the numbers.

that are present when the cancer is diagnosed are one cause of cancer heterogeneity, which makes chemotherapy less effective.

Now let's consider a small population of older, wiser flies that have parented many of the younger, more energetic flies. These older, wiser flies evaded the random fly swats not by being fast or keen-sighted but

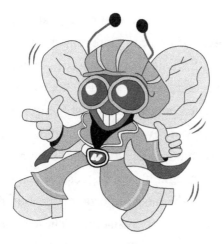

Figure 6.2. Super fly with the ability to evade most flyswatters.

by spending most of their time in the corner, where the ceiling meets two walls. It is not impossible for the flyswatter to get into that corner, but it is incredibly difficult, particularly if the swatting individual is blindfolded. And by squeezing itself into the corner, the fly makes itself nearly invisible, even when the person swatting has no blindfold. Such a "lord of the flies" represents how hard it is to eliminate cancer stem cells, a second cause of cancer heterogeneity.

Why remissions do not translate into cures: Getting to the root of the problem

Producing a partial remission—where cancer is still detectable but the majority of cancer cells have been killed—may improve symptoms if the size or location of the cancer is causing problems for the surrounding normal tissues. As shown in the second figure in the Science Corner on first-order kinetics, however, a partial remission to treatment had little effect on the biology of the cancer. Even a complete remission—meaning the cancer is undetectable—signifies that only

4 logs of cancer cells of the 12 logs present at diagnosis have been eliminated. So even after a complete remission is attained, there is still a lot of work to be done to achieve a cure. Not only are there still lots of cancer cells that need to be killed, but with lots of cancer cells come cancer cell heterogeneity: those fast-flying, keen-sighted, smart super flies that can evade even large flyswatters wielded by unblind-folded individuals and continue to produce even more super flies.

Research by Rick and his colleagues now suggests that cancer stem cells are one of the most important contributors to cancer cell heterogeneity and treatment resistance. These are the older, wiser "lords of the flies" that hide in the corners or, if you prefer, the roots of the dandelion. These cells are hardy, well protected, and hard to find. Since these are the cells that initiate the cancer and are most critical for producing new cancer cells, it is critical to study them, but the difficulty finding them has made it challenging to do so. Accordingly, the development of most anticancer agents has been aimed at the part of the cancer that is easily studied, or the part of the dandelion above the ground. Perhaps not surprisingly, the cancer research community has developed effective therapies for the bulk of the cancer cells, but such therapies often spare the rare cancer stem cells. The fastest way to get rid of the dandelion is to use a lawn mower (figure 6.3), which will quickly and effectively eradicate the visible part of the weed (put the yard into a complete remission). To prevent the weed from regrow-ing, however, the unseen roots also need to be eliminated. Since can-cer researchers have been studying primarily the part of the cancer they can see, there are lots of effective lawn mowers for cancer but few root removers.

Not only are cancer stem cells hard to identify and find, but it is difficult to determine whether a potentially effective treatment works against them. For example, if an anti-weed treatment attacked the root of the dandelion while sparing the visible part of the weed because

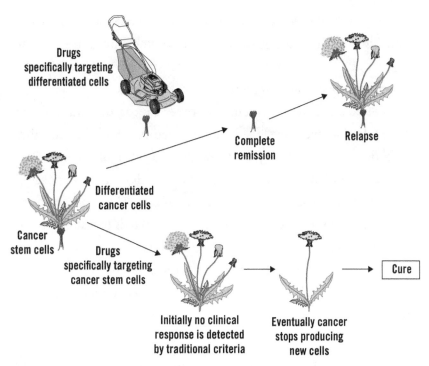

Figure 6.3. How chemotherapy affects cancer stem cells compared with how it affects the cancer cells that make up most of a cancer. The fastest way to get rid of dandelions is to use a lawn mower, which will quickly and effectively eradicate the visible part of the weed—putting the yard into a complete remission. Since cancer researchers have primarily been studying the part of the cancer they can see (the dandelion plant), it is not surprising that the cancer research community has developed highly effective therapies for the bulk of cancer (lawn mowers), but such therapies often miss the rare cancer stem cells (the dandelion root).

it was biologically different, there would be no immediately discernible effect on the weed's flower and leaves. Over time the dandelion would wither and die, but this process would take longer than just cutting it down. Similarly, treatments that specifically attack cancer stem cells will not immediately eliminate cancer. In such a situation, cure (elimination of the cancer stem cells) in effect precedes the clinical demonstration of complete remission (clearance of the bulk cancer cells) and could even occur without actual disease shrinkage. Because waiting for the visible part of the weed to wither takes longer than just mowing it down, it is not surprising that using clinical response to determine the effectiveness of anticancer therapies may miss treatments that specifically target the cancer stem cells.

Let's assume that a potential cure for cancer, including cancer stem cells, has been developed—like a "weed-be-gone" that can eliminate dandelion roots. Digging through the dirt to make sure the root has been eliminated would be pointless since it is nearly impossible to confirm the absence of a small residual root. The only way to tell whether the weed is gone, or the cancer is cured, is to watch to see if it regrows. It is usually held that most cancers will grow back within five years if not cured. This is generally the case, though not always, as cancer stem cells occasionally remain dormant for longer periods of time.

If it can't be cured, can it be controlled? Can cancer be like high blood pressure?

Since the enormous number of cells and their heterogeneity make curing many cancers a formidable task, researchers are studying ways to control cancer as a chronic disease, like high blood pressure or diabetes. While both high blood pressure and diabetes are incurable and occasionally life threatening, neither of these diseases is considered a death sentence. They can be controlled, with most affected patients living fairly normal lives. So can cancer be controlled, just as one might periodically mow the lawn to keep the dandelions down? The answer is: sometimes.

When Rick's young family moved to the suburbs to have a big yard for the kids to play in, they bought a house whose previous owners had a lawn service. Nearly 40 years ago environmental lawn services were not yet in fashion, and most used lots of chemicals. In fact, the previous owner's lawn service was called—somewhat hard to imagine today—ChemLawn. Rick's wife, Lynn, refused to allow the lawn service anywhere near their yard, afraid of the effects of the chemicals on rabbits and squirrels, not to mention kids. For a couple of years, their lawn looked immaculate, like the yard on the left in figure 6.4, but eventually the dandelions made their way back (see the yard on the right). Some would say the lawn needs to be mowed whenever a dandelion pops up, but clearly they'll just grow back. So what's the hurry? After about 10 years, it was impossible to keep the dandelions down, even with weekly mowing. Their solution, since a lawn service was out of the question, was of course to move. Again, they picked a house with a beautiful yard thanks to the previous owners and their lawn service, and the same 10-year dandelion cycle was repeated. By this time the kids had moved out of the house, so Rick and Lynn

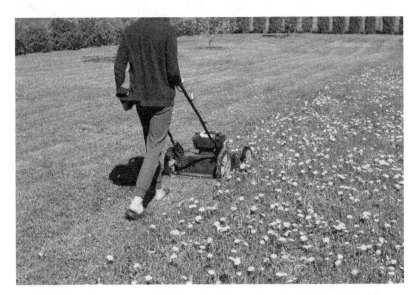

Figure 6.4. What Rick's yard looked like when they moved in (*left*) and moved out (*right*).

moved into a townhouse in Baltimore's Inner Harbor, nearer to Johns Hopkins and with no yard to worry about!

In many ways, controlling cancer is similar to dealing with dandelions in the yard. Many cancers—mostly of the slow-growing, indolent variety—can be effectively controlled just by watching and waiting, with occasional lawn mowing when necessary. This is the general approach for follicular lymphomas, early multiple myeloma, chronic lymphocytic leukemia, and, often, prostate cancer. For these diseases, though they are generally incurable, median survival is measured in decades.

A major component in the long survival achieved with these cancers is limiting chemotherapy or avoiding it altogether. Standard chemotherapy, sometimes called cytotoxic (*cyto* = cell; *toxic* is self-explanatory) chemotherapy, consists of nonspecific poisons that affect all cells, especially those that are rapidly dividing. Not only is cytotoxic chemotherapy harmful to normal organs (just as overmowing and lawn chemicals can damage the grass), but it can also induce additional genetic mutations in cancer cells, causing them to transform into fast-growing, aggressive cancers. Instead, targeted and immunologic therapies are generally called upon when these indolent malignancies need treatment (see chapter 8, "Cancer Treatments"). Such therapies are generally less toxic to normal organs than cytotoxic chemotherapy, as well as less likely to produce genetic damage that could transform the cancer.

Controlling aggressive incurable cancers—most solid organ cancers fall into this category—is much less successful. Even mowing won't control crabgrass for long, because it grows so fast. Moreover, the indolent cancers often eventually transform, like the aggressive dandelions in Rick and Lynn's yard before they moved. Still, controlling cancer for a decade or two is something worth celebrating.

There is one type of cancer where lawn mowing may actually keep the dandelions in check, perhaps life-long: chronic myeloid leukemia, or CML. When Rick's dad was diagnosed with CML in 1970, patients with CML had a median survival of three to four years. Bone marrow transplantation became a cure for CML patients in the 1980s (too late to help his dad), but in the late 1990s, with the development of imatinib (brand name, Gleevec), the disease became like high blood pressure. This drug attacks the genetic mutation that causes CML: the Philadelphia chromosome (named for where it was discovered), or *BCR-ABL*. It launched the era of targeted therapies, expected by many to be the long-awaited "cure" for cancer. In actuality, imatinib usually doesn't cure CML, but it is a highly effective lawn mower, keeping the dandelions down perhaps for as long as it continues to be used.

Although targeted therapies have become useful parts of the cancer treatment arsenal over the past 20 years, they have not been such dramatic successes in other cancers. CML turns out to be a unique cancer in that it is essentially caused by one genetic mutation, *BCR-ABL*, instead of the multiple mutations needed to cause most cancers. Since this is the only mutation that drives the cancer cells, targeting the mutation keeps the cancer completely in check, though it is not lethal to the leukemia. Because all other cancers are driven by multiple mutations, targeting one mutation will not produce the same success as targeting the single mutation behind CML. Occasionally CML presents with additional mutations, a transformed state called blast crisis. In this situation, imatinib will not keep CML in check, and a bone marrow transplant, discussed in chapter 8, is needed to control the blast crisis.

Conclusion: In search of the cure

There will never be a single cure for cancer, since cancer is a myriad of different diseases, all featuring different biology and requiring different therapies. Even treating a single cancer can require different treatments for multiple mutations. The pace of cancer treatment approvals by the FDA has never been faster. These treatments have proven successful in reducing the size of cancers and have led to improved health and quality of life, especially when the cancer interferes with critical functions, as brain cancers do. This alone justifies using a partial remission—at least a 50% reduction in size of the cancer—as a criterion for drug approvals rather than waiting for long-term results.

A partial remission, however, doesn't represent a cure. A complete analysis of treatment impacts requires lots of time and plenty of data to determine long-term gains and possibly identify cures. I asked Rick how this analysis and data gathering are being accomplished and who is doing it.

Long-term treatment impacts are analyzed in several ways. First of all, the collective experience of oncologists is shared within practices and hospitals and through scientific journals and conferences. Ultimately, the impacts of new treatments are analyzed through longitudinal studies, but these are expensive, require years or decades for results, and typically focus on a single cancer. The Surveillance, Epidemiology, and End Results (SEER) Program of the National Cancer Institute collects data on cancer cases from locations and sources throughout the United States. Data collection began in 1973 with a limited number of registries and continues to expand to include even more areas and demographics. Currently, however, there are registries in only 17 states. The International Agency for Research on

Cancer (IARC), part of the World Health Organization, collects and publishes surveillance data on the occurrence of cancer worldwide.

This all sounds good, but as a health care consumer I have to vent a big frustration. Having worked in the field of information technology (IT) for many decades, I am well aware of the challenges of data integration and the associated problems when data silos (when data is known only within a department and not shared and combined with company data) prevent a company from having a complete picture of operational or financial data. Although data integration has gotten better within health care systems and hospitals (there are even some web portals available where you can fill out forms and look stuff up), we all still suffer the frustration of going to a new doctor who knows absolutely nothing about our medical history or, worse, realizing that your heart specialist isn't aware of what your cancer specialist is doing. Unfortunately, the burden of information sharing falls heavily on the patient, and if that patient isn't so well organized, or maybe getting older and forgetful, or maybe can't find the car keys or remember a bloody thing—well, you get the picture.

Wouldn't it be wonderful if cancer doctors could have at their fingertips the long-term patient results of everyone globally who had cancer X and was treated with A, B, and C? Of course, wishing won't make it so. How do we make it so? It's probably too late for me to do anything with my already out-of-date IT background. It is time for our talented children, nieces, and nephews to step up to this challenge.

CHAPTER 7

Diagnosing Cancer

Better the Devil You Know Than the Devil You Don't

SO FAR, I HAVE DESCRIBED how normal and cancer cells grow and behave, debunked some myths about cancer, introduced the cancer stem cell, and explained the mechanisms that allow cancer to spread throughout the body. Before we get into the details of treatment in the next chapter, let's talk about the psychology of finding out that you might have cancer.

The specter of cancer: WTH

You are feeling fine, and you notice something unusual. Maybe a mole on your leg is looking strange. Maybe you feel a new lump in your neck. Maybe you have a pain in your back that can't be explained by too much yoga or a recent Netflix binge. Maybe a woman notices something in her breast. Maybe a man has gotten a high PSA score on a recent blood test. Perhaps something is found as part of a regular screening mammogram or colonoscopy or pops up on an x-ray, CT scan, MRI, or other diagnostic test done for some other reason. This "something" might be called a lump, or a spot, or a lesion, or a mass, or even a tumor (which, by the way, just means a lump, not necessarily cancerous), but it always raises the specter of cancer.

My mom's lung cancer was first noticed—though initially missed until I showed the scan to Rick—on a routine x-ray when she broke her hip. Rick's dad's diagnosis of chronic myeloid leukemia was initially suggested on a routine blood test as part of his annual physical. In any case, when the specter of cancer is raised, it's natural to yell "what the hell!" (figure 7.1). (Most of us would really say "WTF!" but this is a book we hope the whole family might read.)

Denial: Ignore it and it might go away

If the patient is the first one to notice WTH, there might be a strong temptation to ignore it and hope for the best. This is rarely a good

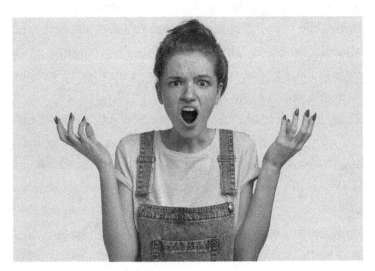

Figure 7.1. Just in case you had any question about what "WTH" stands for.

option. Cancer is never diagnosed early in its course, but that in no way means that a timely diagnosis is unimportant. Yes, by the time cancer is initially diagnosed, it has probably been traveling throughout the bloodstream for a while. To set up shop in a metastatic location, however, circulating cancer cells must gain the ability to grow outside of their usual microenvironment. This is a random occurrence that may or may not have happened by the time of diagnosis. Perhaps most important, the lack of a timely diagnosis can weigh heavily on an individual, both emotionally and physically.

As my name suggests, my heritage is Irish. One of the most famous Irish proverbs says "Better the devil you know than the devil you don't," and nothing could be truer when the specter of cancer is raised. Worrying about whether WTH could be cancer may cause even the most self-confident, unflappable person to go off the rails. In contrast, when patients learn their actual diagnosis instead of having to deal with the unknown, Rick finds that their demeanor often changes in a positive direction. Often, maybe even more often than not, the answer to a biopsy or other test comes back benign. But even when the opposite occurs, patients usually shift gears and are ready to take cancer on. The best time to address cancer is when the patient is in shape to deal with the cancer—before the cancer has had detrimental effects on one's health.

Thus, it is always better to get professional advice if you are dealing with WTH, maybe after you have spent a week going crazy reading Google sites and testimonials. If it's a doctor who first finds WTH as part of a screening or a test done for another reason, you have someone who can immediately give you advice about the next steps and guide you along the way. And this might be the only time in your life that you can get a referral appointment with a specialist quickly.

Getting to a diagnosis: To b(iopsy) or not to b(iopsy), that is the question

Patients typically have many questions when first getting medical help for WTH, starting with, Is WTH cancer or not? If so, what kind of cancer is it? And what is the best way to figure this out? Biopsies are the most common tool to analyze lumps, unusual skin growths, swollen lymph nodes, colon polyps, and so on. So what is the right type of biopsy, and is one even needed (figure 7.2)? Take the man with the high PSA (note: low scores are good, but high PSA scores don't necessarily mean cancer). The usual way to know for sure is fishing around for microscopic cancer cells in the prostate with a biopsy. The same goes for breast lumps and other suspicious "somethings."

Sometimes, particularly with blood cancers, blood tests alone are sufficient to diagnose a cancer. Even solid organ cancers may soon be reliably diagnosed with non-invasive blood tests known as liquid biopsies given that cells from most cancers, even localized ones, circulate to some extent in the bloodstream. Although liquid biopsies are

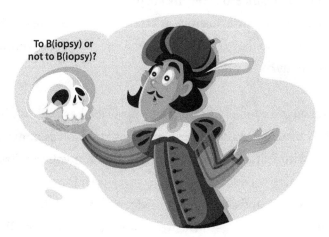

To B(iopsy) or not to B(iopsy)?

Figure 7.2. Hamlet contemplates the age-old question.

still largely in the experimental phase, it is likely that looking for cancer cells or cancer cell DNA in the blood may soon become standard practice.

The right answer on how and when to diagnose WTH may seem crystal clear, but it often isn't as simple as it seems. Sometimes the correct answer is to just observe to see if the WTH changes. Admittedly, this approach would drive many people crazy. In all cases, it is best to put WTH into perspective and think about the big picture. Some important considerations are the following:

- How old are you?
- How is your general health, and do you have any underlying illnesses?
- What are your current symptoms?
- What is your history of cancer, if any?
- What is your family's history of cancer, if any?
- What are the risks of the diagnostic procedure, and will the results be definitive?
- What noncancerous results are possible?
- If the results are cancerous, what types of cancer are most likely, and how do these types of cancer grow and spread throughout the body?

A recommended biopsy might be described as minimally invasive. This usually means a needle biopsy that involves numbing the skin and withdrawing tissue—no fun at all but involving little risk. Getting enough cells for diagnosis may require minor surgery, which is more invasive and poses greater risks. Sometimes, if the lesion is difficult to get to or if less invasive approaches such as needle biopsies are nondiagnostic, major surgery might even be necessary.

A relatively simple, minimally invasive needle biopsy may not be the best approach to getting a diagnosis or may even provide misleading information. While we were writing this book, my wife's sister Paula noticed the dreaded lump in her neck. Paula is never one to shy away from anything, so she immediately contacted her primary doctor, who quickly referred her to an ENT (ear, nose, and throat doctor, or otolaryngologist), who promptly performed a needle biopsy of the neck lymph node. As often occurs with the small samples obtained with needle biopsies, the results came back inconclusive but looking suspicious for lymphoma.

Paula reached out to Rick, who asked her a series of questions: Had she noticed any other symptoms or lumps? The answer was no. Was the lymph node easily movable? Yes. How fast was it growing? She told him it had even gotten a bit smaller. He told her that enlarged lymph nodes are one of the most common "somethings" that lead patients to doctors. It is normal for lymph nodes to swell and shrink—they are the so-called swollen glands associated with colds and sore throats—as white blood cells rush there to fight off infection and then leave as infection goes away. Lots of things cause lymph nodes to enlarge, including pimples, local skin irritation, and even vaccinations. Rick told her that 90% of lymph node biopsies are benign—especially those that are otherwise asymptomatic and not getting bigger—and she should wait about a month to see if it grew. Paula's nature is to attack problems head on, and she had the whole lymph node immediately removed in what is called an excisional biopsy. The good news is that it was completely benign.

Were getting the needle biopsy and then the excisional biopsy the right decisions? Well, getting a prompt diagnosis is probably never the wrong decision. However, the initial needle biopsy was probably not the correct procedure. The preferred procedure for diagnosing lymphoma is an excisional biopsy, and if the node is easily accessible, like one in the neck, under the arm, or in the groin, that procedure should be performed instead of a needle biopsy. Although a bit more invasive, removing a lymph node from under the skin is far from major surgery, and the larger amount of tissue obtainable by removing the entire node makes it the preferred choice. Think of trying to identify your Uncle Joe in a room with hundreds of people by only being able to look at his ears. Although your Uncle Joe may have distinctive ears, it would certainly be easier if you had more information—if you could see the faces of Uncle Joe and all the others.

A failed needle biopsy increases medical costs, can lead to delays in diagnosis, and can produce unnecessary anxiety, as in Paula's case. In fact, lymphoma specialists spend a lot of time trying to convince surgeons that although a needle biopsy may seem like a kinder and gentler procedure, it is preferable to go right to an excisional biopsy for easily accessible lumps. Moreover, in Paula's case, since the lump was stable and even getting smaller in size, waiting at least a month before going to the excisional biopsy may have allowed her to avoid the procedure altogether.

At the same time Paula was going through her WTH ordeal, one of Rick's coworkers, the head transplant case manager at Johns Hopkins, Kathryn, noted enlarged, somewhat painful lymph nodes under her left arm and in her left neck. As she deals with lymphoma patients needing a bone marrow transplant daily, she was worried and frantically called Rick for advice. Two days earlier she had just gotten a Shingrix (shingles) shot in her left arm, but swollen lymph nodes were not listed as a side effect. Rick told her that vaccination is actually a common cause of enlarged lymph nodes. No biopsy was done, and as expected the nodes normalized over a few days.

Paula's and Kathryn's stories both have happy endings, but for Paula and her family the many weeks of worry, tears while expecting

the worst, and pain of a biopsy and surgery were a big strain. Many would consider Paula's experience (a specialist appointment to identify a cancer risk, an initial needle biopsy, an excisional biopsy, and then a diagnosis) to be standard operating procedure, but was this truly the best approach? What if Paula's ENT had initially said (1) this lump is most likely benign, (2) it will probably go away on its own, and (3) let me check again in one month. Are doctors inclined to be overly cautious? Do medical liability risks, insurance reimbursement considerations, or medical specialty silos drive us toward "standard procedures" that miss the mark for the individual? These are probably questions for another book. The bottom line for Paula's story is that more knowledge and perspective provided by a lymphoma specialist (Rick in this case) helped reduce her anxiety and increase her confidence in the steps that were taken.

Let's discuss a couple of other common examples of the decision-making analysis that goes on when diagnosing WTH. Take a man in his mid-40s with a darkened mole and a history of melanoma in his family. He is in good health with no other known cancer. He is examined by a dermatologist, who scrapes some cells and sends these off for analysis. The results come back as pre-melanoma. Even though the diagnosis is benign, he is appropriately scheduled for surgery to remove the mole and test that the margins of skin around the mole are healthy. The risks of the biopsy and surgery are minimal, and the risks of a pre-melanoma becoming actual cancer in the lifetime of a young man is high.

Now imagine the man is in his early 90s with unusual moles that were visually identified as basal cell skin cancer on his arms and neck. He is in poor health, with heart problems, and had been previously treated with chemotherapy for indolent lymphoma, which is stable. Here it is probably not worth taking even the low risk of infection and bleeding associated with minor surgery to remove the moles. The moles aren't causing him any problem, and thus removing them won't add to his quality of life. A similar risk-benefit ratio exists for a woman in her 90s with an asymptomatic small lymph node under her arm that has been growing slowly for several years. Unlike Paula's lymph node, this one is not likely to be benign, given its long history, but with slow growth, it is likely an indolent lymphoma that would not require treatment. And remember, the patient is in her 90s!

These relatively simplistic examples illustrate the key point that early on it is important to talk through all these questions with your doctor. Sometimes the diagnosis can be made just by simple inspection—such as in the case of a benign mole or a small lymph node that isn't growing—and other times it is best to observe what happens over a short period of time, like a month or so. In other scenarios, such as when a lymph node is growing rapidly or a mole looks funny, a timely biopsy may be needed. There may be times when your doctor can't answer the questions, and then it is important to take the time to find a cancer specialist and discuss options with that person.

OK, I have cancer—now what? On your mark, get set, go

What if Paula's biopsy had come back positive for cancer? In many if not most patients, the anxiety actually fades after a definitive diagnosis of cancer is made. Energy naturally shifts toward action and the push to deal with a "known" health challenge. However, in some patients a diagnosis of cancer worsens anxiety and even produces profound depression. Although some degree of the blues is understandable with getting such news, the reality is that cancer is no longer a death sentence. Many patients won't even need treatment for indolent disease, many other patients are now cured, and many more will be curable in the near future with new and emerging therapies.

Even when not curable, most cancers can now be controlled for some period of time. There are lots of resources for both dealing with the shock of the diagnosis and for answering the myriad questions that will initially be running through the mind of every patient diagnosed with cancer. These questions will include the following:

- How does this cancer typically progress, and what are the best- and worst-case scenarios?
- How much has my cancer progressed?
- What damage has the cancer already caused, and how is this impacting my health?
- Do I have any symptoms?
- Where is the cancer likely to spread, and are there any indications of this yet?
- What are the treatment options for the primary cancer site?
- What are the treatment options to prevent or slow the cancer's spread?

Where can you get help and find answers? Although your family and friends may have well-intended opinions about what to do next, I suggest taking their guidance with a grain of salt unless one of them is an oncologist like Rick. The Internet is another potential source of both wisdom and, unfortunately, misinformation. Reliable sources include the National Cancer Institute, the American Cancer Society, the National Comprehensive Cancer Network, and a variety of disease foundation websites, which offer useful links to other reputable sources of information about specific cancers (see Online Resources at the end of this book). But regardless of how much information you gather on your own, it is now time to see an oncologist.

If we can make a running analogy, which Paula happens to love, all these prior steps are about getting ready for "the run" (figure 7.3).

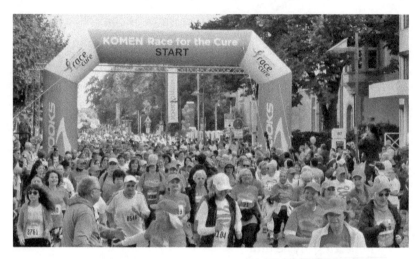

Figure 7.3. Starting the Susan G. Komen Race for the Cure. (*Source:* Wikimedia Commons, CC-BY-SA-3.0.)

You have decided what to do, and now the run, or treatment, begins. Maybe your run is an easy walk in the park (also called watchful waiting), and no specific treatment is needed. Maybe your run is the beginning of a marathon, starting with major surgery like the Whipple procedure for pancreatic cancer, which removes the head of the pancreas, the first part of the small intestine (duodenum), the gallbladder, and the bile duct. At a minimum, continual monitoring or watching will be part of the run.

In all cases, this is just the beginning of the run. Additional treatments and therapies may be part of the run, each with decisions to be made and risks to be weighed. Taking the time to ask questions and to understand the options with your oncologist is the key to making the best of your run. And it goes without saying that you should ask for the support of your friends and family before, during, and after the run. It is easier to run a long race with crowds cheering along the route.

CHAPTER 8

Cancer Treatments

Winning the Battle without Losing the War

HOPEFULLY, IT IS BECOMING CLEAR why cancer remains so difficult to cure: not only are there billions and billions of heterogeneous cancer cells present at diagnosis, but they've learned how to be invisible to the immune system, arise from hardy stem cells that live in protected microenvironments, and move around a lot. The good news, however, is that there also has been substantial progress, especially since the turn of the millennium, in improving the outcomes of cancer patients even when they can't be cured.

As already discussed, some cancers, such as many follicular lymphomas and prostate cancers, are so slow growing that patients can live for decades without much therapy. In these cancers, a do-no-harm approach is generally taken since cure is difficult or not yet possible and treatment can cause its own problems, maybe even helping the cancer transform into a more aggressive form. Since the treatment for these slow-growing cancers is not curative and can actually be worse than the disease, it is generally avoided until there are symptoms requiring therapy. Other cancers, such as chronic myeloid leukemia and multiple myeloma, are not curable but can, like high blood pressure or diabetes, be controlled with therapy, often for decades. For some cancers, especially many solid organ cancers such as pancreatic cancer, the goal of treatment—often surgery or radiation—is to prolong life by relieving symptoms and keeping the body functioning. Even a cure is becoming increasingly plausible for many cancers.

This chapter will discuss the various forms of therapy used to lessen symptoms, control cancer, or even cure it. The focus will be on general concepts rather than specific treatments for specific cancers since these treatments are continuously changing for the better. The concepts underpinning treatments, however, don't change. One key principle is that the treatment should not be worse than the disease. The medical community has learned the hard way that sometimes the toxicity of treatment outweighs any benefit. Since many cancer treatments are poisons (arsenic is an obvious example), it is not surprising that most cancer therapies have serious side effects. Weighing the benefits versus the risks is central to determining the best approach to dealing with an individual's specific cancer. For aggressive life-threatening cancers, an all-out battle with associated casualties (that is, side effects) to win the war usually needs to be waged. For other slow-growing, indolent cancers, winning an early battle with the disease could lead to losing the overall war, since treatment can sometimes make the cancer worse by inducing additional mutations.

Attacking cancer while avoiding normal cells

For a treatment to be no worse than the cancer being treated, the following simplistic equation should be true: the number of cancer cells killed is greater than the number of normal cells killed. This equation has bothered me since we started writing this book, and it reminds me of an old joke about how a thermos is able to keep both cold things cold and hot things hot—how do it know? (figure 8.1). Since most cancer treatments have essentially nonspecific effects on all cells—surgery, radiation, and most chemotherapies cannot distinguish cancer cells from normal cells—why are they more active against cancer than against normal cells?

Surgical treatments remove both cancerous masses and the margins of normal tissue. To minimize the healthy tissue that is removed, Mohs surgery for skin cancer, for example, tests surgically removed samples incrementally. After surgical removal of a skin cancer, usually under local anesthesia in a doctor's office, the specimen is examined under a microscope for cancerous cells. If cancer is found, the surgeon goes back and removes the indicated cancerous tissue from the patient. This procedure is repeated until no further microscopic cancer is found.

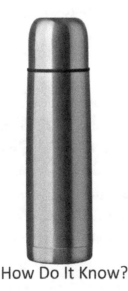

How Do It Know?

Figure 8.1. The ability of chemotherapy to distinguish between cancer and normal cells is a bit like the brilliance of a thermos in keeping cold things cold and hot things hot.

Radiation therapy uses high-energy particles or waves to kill cancer cells and as few healthy cells as possible. In an attempt to limit the damage to normal cells, sophisticated radiation planning and delivery techniques are employed. Today, with such inventions as CyberKnife radiation and proton beam therapy, treatment can be tightly targeted, further limiting the damage to healthy cells.

Chemotherapy drugs are essentially nonspecific poisons that affect all cells, cancerous and normal. The mechanisms associated with chemotherapy and "how it knows" to attack primarily the cancer cells are complicated and will be explored later. Finally, targeted therapies, as the name implies, are specifically designed to mess with critical cancer cellular functions, but these same functions are often present in normal cells.

Before digging into the details of treatment options, let's review the challenges that successful therapies must meet using Rick's favorite gardening analogies. Imagine you bought a new home and want to revive the lawn and flower beds, which have not been tended to for some time, as a parallel to starting treatment for a new diagnosis of cancer.

1. *First, get rid of the rocks.* Before planting a beautiful lawn or flower bed, you need to get rid of the rocks or the grass and flowers won't grow. To eliminate symptoms and sometimes just to stay alive, some cancers must be removed through surgery or shrunken through targeted radiation.

2. *Next, get rid of the weeds and pests.* Getting rid of weeds and pests in the lawn and in flower gardens is hard work and can have untoward effects. Removing them by hand, one by one, is impractical. Pesticides and weed killers do kill weeds but can also damage the grass and flowers and harm the environment. Sometimes, if the dandelion flowers and colorful bugs

are not doing too much harm, they can just be enjoyed. Chemotherapy has to balance the gain in controlling cancer with the harm to healthy tissues.

3. *Finally, target the roots.* Dandelion roots are commonly 6 to 18 inches long and can penetrate to a depth of 10 feet, making it virtually impossible to dig them out. Another approach is to use poisons that will kill the entire plant but inflict collateral damage on other plants and grass. If a special biological or chemical treatment that only disrupted dandelion root growth was applied to a lawn—maybe injected into the soil with a roller or hand sprayed onto the leaves of the dandelion—this would be the equivalent of a targeted cancer treatment. Alternatively, removing some or all of the underlying soil with a backhoe and either replacing the soil or treating it to make it dandelion unfriendly would be the equivalent of a bone marrow transplant.

Local treatments (surgery and radiation): Like a knife through melted butter

Up until the middle of the last century, surgery and radiation were the only options for treating cancer. Surgery for cancer has been around for millennia, with the first description of mastectomy for breast cancer dating from AD 200. The use of radiation for cancer followed only a couple years after the initial discovery of x-rays by Wilhelm Roentgen in 1895. Both surgery and radiation can remove visible cancers, even large ones, and are therefore highly effective at reducing harmful local effects of cancer masses. Brain cancers are prime examples where surgery, radiation, or both are critical, even though not curative. These cancers take up space in a constricted area and can wreak havoc by increasing pressure in the brain as well as damaging normal brain cells and nerves that no longer have room to function. Radiation can also be highly effective in reducing the local effects of lymphomas and other cancers. Improvements in surgical techniques, including minimally invasive, image-guided laparoscopic procedures, have also made it possible to remove small growths with minimal risk.

Yet surgery and radiation are usually not able to get it all, as the cancer often has spread by the time it is diagnosed. Essentially all blood cancers have spread by the time they are diagnosed, since moving around is what their normal counterparts do. Although nonblood cancers are often called solid organ cancers, they also usually become blood-borne (or take liquid form) months or even years before they can be diagnosed (as discussed in chapter 4 on metastases). So Rick suggests that surgery and radiation, instead of being able to remove cancer "like a hot knife through butter," are like trying to remove cancer "like a knife through *melted* butter" (figure 8.2). Because most cancers have already spread around like melted butter, they can no longer be extracted with the knife.

Attempting to use surgery or radiation to remove microscopic or undetectable disease has a long track record. It was standard practice to make wide surgical incisions around visible cancers hoping to get any unseen "melted butter" that had spread locally. Removal of lymph

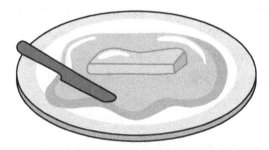

Figure 8.2. A knife attempting to cut melted butter. Since most cancers, even solid organ cancers, have spread like melted butter by the time of diagnosis, a surgical (or radiation) knife alone is unlikely to be curative.

nodes in the region of the original cancer was also common practice in an attempt to eliminate cancer that had spread to draining lymph nodes before it could metastasize further. But because most cancers have already metastasized through the blood by the time they are diagnosed, attempts to cure cancer by surgically removing potential sites of spread have been largely unsuccessful. (Regional lymph node removal is still used diagnostically to assess the risk that the cancer has metastasized.)

Radiation beyond the primary cancer site to treat microscopic disease was a mainstay of treatment for lymphoma, particularly Hodgkin lymphoma, until the turn of this century. Hodgkin lymphoma was thought to spread through the lymphatic system to nearby lymph nodes. This understanding led to radiation treatments called total nodal irradiation (radiating all the lymph nodes in the body) and mantle irradiation (named for the garment, similar to a cloak, and radiating all the lymph nodes in the top half of the body). These radiation strategies for eliminating microscopic disease in lymphomas are rarely performed today, not only because of the toxicity of such extensive radiation but also because chemotherapy can be more effective at getting to the microscopic disease throughout the body.

Surgical and radiation treatments for cancer are associated with substantial risks, some even life threatening. In addition to the risks of the surgery itself—issues related to anesthesia, bleeding, and infection—surgery can damage normal tissues. An example is lymphedema of the arm following lymph node dissection for breast cancer. Lymphedema is the accumulation of fluid in the arm that can occur when surgery disrupts the normal flow of lymphatic fluid between lymph nodes, preventing the fluid from being able to flow out of the arm properly. This condition can cause significant discomfort, increase the risk of skin infections, and sometimes be permanent. Radiation can also damage normal organs, causing lung fibrosis, coronary artery disease, and serious inflammation of the gastrointestinal tract, as well as give rise to secondary cancers.

Both radiation and chemotherapy kill normal and cancer cells by damaging their DNA, but following the principle that "what doesn't kill us makes us stronger," the DNA damage can actually strengthen cancer cells. Studies have found that radiation can induce second cancers more often than chemotherapy does, with up to a 20-fold increased risk of second cancers depending on the age of the patient at treatment. Newer surgical and radiation techniques, including abandoning the extensive surgeries and radiation fields thought necessary in the past, have certainly lessened some of the toxicities of these treatments but do not prevent them entirely.

Cytotoxic chemotherapy: Two heads are better than one, three better than two . . .

The history of successful cytotoxic chemotherapy—the official term for what we commonly call chemotherapy—starts with the treatment of childhood acute lymphoblastic leukemia (ALL), which also arguably remains the field's biggest success story. The story begins with Dr. Sidney Farber, often called the father of modern chemotherapy. ALL is the most common cancer in children and was uniformly and rapidly fatal—often within weeks—through the middle of the twentieth century. Farber, with colleagues around the world, found several effective chemotherapy drugs against ALL, but when only one drug was used the disease would always return. By the turn of the twenty-first century, because of the gradual addition of a second chemotherapy drug and then a third and eventually a fourth, nearly 90% of children with this disease, which had been fatal within weeks half a century earlier, could now expect to be cured.

SCIENCE CORNER

Dr. Sidney Farber and Combination Chemotherapy

Following graduation from Harvard Medical School in 1927, Sidney Farber studied pathology at Peter Bent Brigham Hospital (the predecessor of Brigham and Women's Hospital in Boston). In 1929 he joined the faculty of Harvard Medical School and was appointed the first full-time pathologist at Boston Children's Hospital. His research focused on diseases, especially leukemia, in infants and children.

Acute lymphoblastic leukemia (ALL), the most common cancer in children, was uniformly and rapidly fatal—often within weeks—through the middle part of the twentieth century. Farber discovered that vitamin B_9, also known as folic acid or folate, played a key role in the growth of ALL cells. This finding led him to hypothesize that blocking the function of folic acid might be useful in treating this leukemia. In 1947 he conducted a clinical trial using the folic acid antagonist aminopterin in 16 children with ALL, 10 of whom eventually went into remission. Although all the children eventually relapsed and died, this work was a breakthrough in cancer therapy, showing for the first time that drugs can be effective against leukemia.

Farber's findings were quickly followed by studies showing that several other drugs could produce transient responses (in other words, temporary remissions) when given alone to children with ALL. These drugs included 6-mercaptopurine (6-MP), which was designed to interfere with DNA synthesis, and corticosteroids, which were newly discovered and being tried for essentially every known disease.

Because of the relative rarity of childhood ALL, researchers from several institutions joined together to form clinical trial groups to study this new field of chemotherapy. In the early 1950s the first clinical trials to test combinations of chemotherapy drugs—methotrexate (another folic acid antagonist), corticosteroids, and 6-MP—against childhood ALL were carried out. The children getting these chemotherapy drug combinations lived longer, but all still died, usually within a year.

Because ALL tended to come back in the fluid around the brain and spinal cord, a major advance was made by aggressively treating this cerebrospinal fluid with radiation, drugs, or both, markedly decreasing relapses in these sites. Ultimately, through careful sequential clinical trials, one-half of children were able to be cured of ALL by

(continued)

the early 1970s. Additional clinical trials of drug combinations in childhood ALL continued, and by the turn of the century, nearly 90% of children with this disease—which had been fatal within weeks just 50 years earlier—could now expect to be cured.

In addition to the clinical trial groups put together to study rare cancers like ALL, clinical trial groups were established to study most cancers, both in the United States and internationally. Even common cancers, like lung, colon, breast, and prostate cancers, often require thousands of patients to test potential new therapies. These clinical trials groups are still active today, playing important roles in the development of new cancer treatments.

The realization that two drugs were better than one, three better than two, and four usually better than three led to combination cytotoxic chemotherapy clinical trials over the past half century in virtually every type of cancer. This approach has led to some remarkable successes but with some limitations:

- The majority of patients with aggressive lymphomas (Hodgkin lymphoma, diffuse large B-cell lymphoma, and Burkitt lymphoma) are now cured.
- The vast majority of men with testicular cancer are also now cured.
- By reducing cancer, cytotoxic chemotherapy improves survival and quality of life for most other cancers but doesn't usually provide a cure. Even ALL in older adults is rarely cured with combinations of cytotoxic chemotherapy.

So let's go back to the question regarding chemotherapy: "How do it know?" How does chemotherapy, which is a combination of nonspecific poisons, kill more cancer cells than normal cells? There are three general ways that chemotherapy can kill cancer while avoiding damaging too many normal cells.

1. Chemotherapy is particularly effective when cancer cells are growing faster than normal cells (fast-growing cancers that are curable). Other organs whose cells are not dividing much (bone, heart, and brain) are resistant to most chemotherapies, so collateral damage is limited.

2. Chemotherapy has limited effectiveness when cancer cells receiving anti-apoptotic signals refuse to die, as in the incurable categories of cancers described previously. However, even when cancer cells grow more slowly than normal cells and don't die, those cancer cells may be more dependent on certain signaling pathways than normal cells are, so drugs affecting these pathways will be more active in the cancer cells than in the normal cells. A prime example is the reliance of some cancers on the cell survival (or anti-apoptotic) signal Bcl-2. Although BCL-2 is a normal gene, many cancers like low-grade lymphomas are much more reliant on it than normal cells, allowing them to outlive normal cells. Targeting Bcl-2, as the recently approved drug venetoclax does, will therefore cause cancer cells to die faster than normal cells.

3. When a treatment affects cancer and normal cells to the same degree, there is often a larger reservoir of normal stem cells than cancer stem cells, so killing the same number of cells in each category leaves behind a reservoir of normal stem cells for cell maintenance. An example is the effect of chemotherapy on normal lymphocytes and lymphoma cells. If chemotherapy completely kills lymphoma cells and all the normal

lymphocytes, the latter will grow back from the primitive hematopoietic stem cell.

Targeted therapy: The magic bullet

Targeted therapies, also called molecularly targeted therapies, are anticancer agents that block the growth of cancer cells by interfering
with specific molecules—the molecular targets—needed for the
growth and survival of the cancer. In the broadest sense, all anticancer drugs could meet this definition since they interfere with critical
molecular targets. Ideally, however, therapies target critical molecules
that are expressed in specific cancers and not in normal cells—so-
called magic bullets for cancer (figure 8.3). Targeted therapy forms
the basis for so-called personalized or precision medicine: cancer

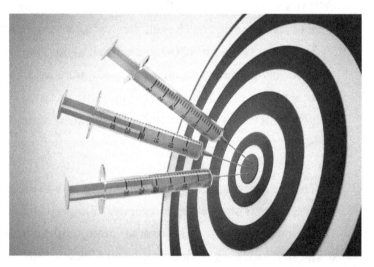

Figure 8.3. The promise of targeted therapy. Although targeted therapies are
revolutionizing how cancer is treated and are often much less toxic than classic
cytotoxic chemotherapy, they are rarely if ever curative as single agents. It is likely,
however, that with more studies and research, these agents will become part of
multipronged attacks that can actually cure many cancers.

treatments tailored to the individual characteristics of each patient and their specific cancer.

Enormous progress has been made in the past two decades with the development of scores of targeted therapies for cancer, but in point of fact there is no such thing as truly specific anticancer therapy. Many of the molecules that are important to cancers are similarly important to normal cells. Many of the genes that cause lymphomas—such as BCL-2 in indolent lymphomas or MYC in aggressive lymphomas—are genes that normal cells also use to grow and survive; they are just overexpressed in the cancer. Thus, targeting such molecules would be expected to also affect normal cells. Even when a molecule is present only in the cancer—such as a genetic mutation that is specific to a cancer, like BCR-ABL in chronic myeloid leukemia—the agent that is developed to target that mutation is almost never perfectly specific for that abnormal molecule and will have some effects on normal molecules. Although targeted therapies are revolutionizing how cancer is treated and are often much less toxic than classic cytotoxic chemotherapy, they are rarely if ever curative as single agents. It is likely, however, that with more studies and research, these agents will become part of multipronged attacks that can eventually cure many cancers.

In the Science Corner on targeted therapies, we've highlighted four examples of targeted therapies and described how they work, their effectiveness, and their limitations:

- drugs that target hormone signaling
- all-trans-retinoic acid (ATRA)—the biologically active form of vitamin A
- monoclonal antibodies—made by cloning white blood cells—that target antigens (proteins) on the surface of cancer cells
- drugs that target specific cancer mutations

SCIENCE CORNER

Targeted Therapies

The development of imatinib in the 1990s to target *BCR-ABL*, or the Philadelphia chromosome, is often heralded as launching the era of targeted therapy. However, the search for targeted therapies actually dates back to more than a century ago.

In the late 1880s it was first suggested, and later shown, that removal of the ovaries, or oophorectomy, could induce remissions in women with breast cancer, but the high mortality associated with the procedure led doctors to essentially abandon it as a treatment in the early 1900s. Studies in the latter part of the twentieth century showed that, contrary to general opinion at the time, oophorectomy offers long-term benefits for patients with breast cancer, including improved survival, returning the procedure to common practice as treatment for the disease. These studies proved that interrupting hormone signaling, which occurs when ovaries producing estrogen and progesterone are removed, could control the growth of cancer. These results formed the basis for the now widespread use of tamoxifen and other anti-estrogens as treatments for breast cancer and anti-androgens as treatments for prostate cancer. Like many targeted therapies, these drugs do not specifically attack cancer but affect all cells, including cancer cells, that need sex hormones for their growth.

Another paradigm of targeted therapy is all-trans-retinoic acid (ATRA) in the treatment of a type of acute myeloid leukemia (AML) called acute promyelocytic leukemia (or APL); this advance also preceded the development of imatinib. ATRA, the biologically active form of vitamin A, is required for the growth of most normal cells. It helps normal stem cells mature or differentiate into mature blood cells. Because cancer cells do not mature normally, many investigators during the second half of the twentieth century began to study whether agents such as ATRA could encourage cancers to grow more normally. Unfortunately, the results of these studies were somewhat disappointing, except for one type of cancer, APL. The first APL patient treated with ATRA was a five-year-old girl treated at the Shanghai Children's Hospital in 1985 after failing standard anti-leukemia therapy. This case was followed by a report from China on the use of ATRA alone in 24 APL patients, with a remarkable complete remission rate of more than 90%. This approach was slow to catch on in the United States and Europe—ATRA wasn't real chemotherapy, after all—and most patients eventually relapsed.

Although it was not known in the 1980s when ATRA was being developed for APL, ATRA is in fact a targeted therapy for this disease. APL is caused by a genetic mutation that is a translocation involving the receptor for ATRA on chromosome 15. Eventually large studies in the mid-1990s demonstrated that ATRA combined with standard anti-leukemia chemotherapy could cure most patients with APL. Now more than 90% of patients with APL are cured without any classic cytotoxic chemotherapy, by combining ATRA with arsenic (yes, arsenic, either with or without old lace).

Another class of targeted therapies are monoclonal antibodies that target markers (or antigens) on cancer cells. Antibodies are made by plasma cells (and sometimes their parents, B lymphocytes) and act like guided missiles, seeking out and destroying unwanted invaders, especially infections. In the 1970s and 1980s, technology was developed for producing antibodies that target specific antigens in the laboratory. This technology continues to be refined, such that monoclonal antibodies against almost any target antigen can now easily be produced. These monoclonal antibodies are routinely armed with various cell poisons, including drugs and radiation—like guided missiles carrying a nuclear payload—to better eliminate their targets.

The first monoclonal antibody approved was rituximab in 1997. Rituximab targets a protein called CD20 on cancerous B lymphocytes and is now used in the treatment of most lymphomas. Just as chemotherapy often isn't specific to cancer cells, rituximab also kills normal B lymphocytes because they also express CD20. However, killing normal B lymphocytes is not a death sentence, since they are remade from stem cells, and even if they weren't, antibodies can be replaced fairly easily.

There are now nearly 100 monoclonal antibodies approved for cancer therapy, including trastuzumab, which targets *HER2*, one of the most important targets in breast cancer, and cetuximab, which targets the epidermal growth receptor present in many solid organ cancers. Because antibodies are produced by the immune system and

(continued)

act by stimulating the immune system, they can also be considered forms of immunotherapy. In practice, the terms "immunotherapy" and "targeted therapy" are often used interchangeably for many forms of immunotherapy.

What most practitioners in the field mean when using the term "targeted therapy" are small molecules that target specific mutations in cancers. This is the class of targeted drugs that imatinib ushered in when it was approved to treat CML in 2002. If monoclonal antibodies are considered guided missiles, these drugs represent jamming signals that disable communication networks within the cancer cells. There are at present nearly 50 approved drugs in this category. It is now common to use molecular testing (also known as next genome sequencing or NGS) on newly diagnosed cancers to look for targetable genetic mutations that may be present in an individual cancer.

Immunotherapy: Reawakening the sleeping giant

Immunotherapy uses the natural power of the immune system to fight cancer. The immune system is a network of cells that work together to protect the body from disease, including infections and cancer. This protection is called immunity. White blood cells, also called leukocytes (from *leuko*, Greek for white), are produced and stored throughout the body. The leukocytes circulate throughout the body between the organs and lymph nodes via the blood and lymphatics. In this way, the immune system works in a coordinated manner to monitor the body for germs or substances that might cause problems and fights back when invaded.

The immune system plays a key role in preventing cancer, in slowing the progress of the disease when it occurs, and in maintaining health during cancer treatments, though the role of natural immunities in preventing cancer is still being researched and debated.

SCIENCE CORNER

The Immune System

There are two basic types of white blood cells: (1) phagocytes, which chew up invading organisms, and (2) lymphocytes, which remember and recognize previous invaders in order to destroy them should they reappear. Several different cells are considered phagocytes. The most common type is the neutrophil (also called a granulocyte), which primarily fights bacteria. Doctors worried about a bacterial infection might order a blood test to see if a patient has an increased number of neutrophils triggered by the infection. Other types of phagocytes, such as monocytes and macrophages, also help the body respond appropriately to specific types of invaders.

The three kinds of lymphocytes are B lymphocytes or B cells, T lymphocytes or T cells, and natural killer cells or NK cells. B cells and their children (plasma cells), which produce antibodies, are like the body's military intelligence system, seeking out their targets and sending defenses to lock onto them. T cells and NK cells are the soldiers, destroying the invaders that the intelligence system has identified.

In the simplest sense, the immune system recognizes not only infections but also cancer cells as foreign and fights to keep them in check. Here's how it works. When antigens (unwanted substances that invade the body) are detected, several types of cells work together to recognize them and respond. B cells are enlisted to produce antibodies, which are specialized proteins that lock onto specific antigens. Once enlisted, these B cells stay in a person's body so that if the immune system encounters that antigen again, the antibodies will be there to do their job. So if someone encounters a disease like measles, that person usually won't get sick from it a second time.

Although antibodies can recognize an antigen and lock onto it, they are not capable of destroying it without help. That's the job of the T cells, which destroy antigens that have been tagged by antibodies or cells that have been infected or somehow changed (like cancer). Antibodies can also neutralize toxins (poisonous or damaging substances) produced by different organisms. Lastly, antibodies can activate a group of proteins called the complement system, which assists in killing bacteria, viruses, or infected cells.

There are two broad types of T cells: cytotoxic T cells that kill and helper T cells that help signal other cells (like phagocytes) to do their jobs. NK cells can attack cells infected by a virus within a few hours or days, and thus can be considered the first line of defense before there is precise recognition of invaders by B and T cells. NK cells can also attack cells that have become cancerous.

Immunotherapy to fight cancer includes several possible approaches. It may involve stimulating your own immune system to work harder or smarter to attack cancer cells. It may entail manipulating the immune system with components designed and manufactured in the laboratory either to better kill cancer cells or to make them more vulnerable to the body's natural defenses. Or it may involve giving a cancer patient a whole new immune system through bone marrow or stem cell transplants.

If the immune system is so strong and sophisticated, why does it fail so often in fighting cancer? There are uncommon situations in which the immune system does not work properly and thus fails as a cancer surveillance system (these occur, for example, when people have HIV/AIDS, hereditary immunodeficiency, or treatment with immunosuppressive drugs for autoimmune diseases). Except for these special situations, cancer often progresses even though the immune system is working normally. Cancers, it turns out, are incredibly cunning in their ability to hide from, avoid, deceive, and occasionally overwhelm the immune system.

Cancers have many ways of avoiding recognition by the immune system. Whatever the exact mechanism by which cancers are able to evade the immune system, they all take advantage of a normal process that controls the immune system called immunologic tolerance. Immunologic tolerance is a complicated process by which the developing immune system is taught to ignore markers on normal cells. Without immunologic tolerance, the immune system may perceive markers on normal cells as unwanted invaders. Autoimmune diseases, or what we might consider "friendly fire," do occur on occasion, but they would occur much more commonly—perhaps every time the immune system gets fired up to fight an infection—if not for immunologic tolerance. Below are three of the major ways that cancers evade the immune system:

1. Some cancers, especially many lymphomas, do not express abnormal proteins but rather go haywire because they express too much of a normal protein that will not be recognized as dangerous by the immune system. This is the case for Burkitt lymphoma, which results from overexpression of the normal Myc protein, and follicular lymphomas, which are caused by overexpression of normal Bcl-2 (see the Science Corner on the genetics of lymphoma in chapter 5).

2. Many of the abnormal mutated genes that cause cancer look like the normal genes they arose from and are thus ignored by the immune system. For example, *BCR-ABL*, the abnormal gene formed by the gene translocation that causes chronic myelogenous leukemia (CML) and some forms of acute lymphoblastic leukemia (ALL), does not stimulate the normal immune system to attack.

3. Even if the initial genetic mutation causing the cancer is invisible to the immune system, many additional mutations that could be recognized develop as cancers grow from one to nearly a trillion cells. However, cancers can turn off markers on cancer cells that the immune system uses to attack the cancer, as well as produce substances that paralyze the immune system, or "put it to sleep."

Nevertheless, it has been clear for decades that the immune system can cure even fully established cancer (see the next section on bone marrow transplantation). Despite hints in animal models and many human trials, immunotherapy for cancer showed little clinical activity (outside of bone marrow transplants) in patients until the past decade. Recently, several different approaches showed it was possible to reawaken the sleeping immune system and arm it against cancer.

In general, five broad immunotherapy approaches are currently being used clinically:

1. *Monoclonal antibodies* target specific markers on cancer cells.
2. *Armed monoclonal antibodies* strengthen antibodies to kill cancer cells.
3. *Immune checkpoint inhibitors* reawaken the immune system to attack cancer cells.
4. *Adoptive cell therapy* uses T cells and NK cells, often after improving on their numbers and function in the laboratory, to better fight cancer.
5. *CAR T cells,* perhaps the ultimate immunologic weapon against cancer, are T cells grown or engineered to specifically recognize a cancer target.
6. *Bispecific antibodies* are manufactured to recognize both cancer cells and the soldiers of the immune system, T cells, thus bringing the T cells directly to where they are needed.

There are several other approaches to enhancing the immune system's innate ability to treat cancer, but most have not yet generated much clinical benefit. One approach has garnered extensive publicity and so deserves some mention: cancer vaccines. Cancer vaccines are analogous to vaccinations against infections—they use proteins from the cancer or inactivated cancer cells themselves to stimulate the immune system to fight the cancer. However, standard vaccines work by stimulating the immune system to recognize the infection before it occurs and are generally ineffective if given for the first time after a full-blown infection has developed. Similarly, cancer vaccines that are given after the cancer has fully developed would not be expected to be able to reawaken an immune system at a time when it is tolerant of the cancer. And since there are thousands of cancers, it would be impossible to immunize patients for all of them.

SCIENCE CORNER

Immunotherapies

Monoclonal antibodies aid the immune system by prompting NK cells to target specific markers (or antigens) on cancer cells. *Armed monoclonal antibodies* are targeted therapies that strengthen antibodies with a bigger killing payload. Most new immunotherapies enhance the activity of T cells along with their close relatives, NK cells, the immune system's soldiers that look to destroy invaders, including cancer, in the body.

Immune checkpoint inhibitors perhaps best highlight the role of the immune system in cancer surveillance and treatment. Immune checkpoints, the targets of this therapy, are key regulators of T cells. When these checkpoints are stimulated, they essentially put the T cells to sleep. This is a crucial component of normal immunologic tolerance that prevents the immune system from attacking normal cells. Some cancer cells can prevent the immune system from attacking them by producing substances that stimulate these immune checkpoint targets. Immune checkpoint inhibitors disable these checkpoints and reawaken or energize the soldiers.

The first anticancer immune checkpoint inhibitor drug approved in the United States was the monoclonal antibody ipilimumab, which was authorized for treatment of melanoma in 2011. The FDA has now approved six immune checkpoint inhibitors for cancer treatment, with more on the way. These drugs are most active against cancers with many mutations that can be seen and attacked by T cells, a characteristic of many solid organ cancers. Blood cancers generally have fewer such mutations and tend to be less responsive to immune checkpoint inhibition. An exception to this rule is Hodgkin lymphoma, which is exquisitely responsive to checkpoint inhibitors. Although these drugs show impressive activity against cancers that are resistant to other therapies, they are rarely curative when used as the sole therapy. Immune checkpoint inhibitors break immune tolerance not only against cancer cells but also against normal cells, leading occasionally to serious, and in rare cases even fatal, autoimmunity.

(continued)

If energizing the soldiers is one effective immunotherapy, another is to make them better fighters, through either better training or better weapons. This is the strategy behind *adoptive cell therapy*, which essentially consists of removing T (or NK) cells from patients with cancer, teaching them in the laboratory to better fight the cancer, and then giving them back. There are several strategies for doing this. One approach is to culture the T cells with proteins present on the cancer to both increase T-cell numbers and make them more active against the cancer. Another strategy is to genetically engineer the T cells to give them better weapons; this is the concept behind *chimeric antigen receptor (or CAR) T cells*. These T cells are chimeric (from the chimera of Greek mythology with a lion's head, a goat's body, and a serpent's tail) in that they combine the soldiering function of a T cell with the guided missile activity of a monoclonal antibody.

CAR T cells can be thought of as the ultimate warrior against cancer, producing remissions and occasionally even cures when all else has failed. However, as one might expect of such powerful treatments, they also have significant negative side effects. CAR T cells can lay waste to not only their cancer targets but also innocent bystanders. The target of a CAR T cell must be specific to the cancer, or, if the target is also expressed by normal cells, those normal cells must be nonessential to the body. Since most cancer targets also appear on normal cells, it has been difficult to find appropriate targets for CAR T cells.

Currently, the only approved CAR T cell therapies are those that target B-cell antigens: CD19 on the cancerous B cells in lymphomas and B lymphocytic leukemias, and BCMA on multiple myeloma. These markers, like CD20, the target of rituximab, are also on normal B cells and plasma cells. Thus, these CAR T cells, like rituximab, also kill normal B cells. Fortunately, B cells and their children's plasma cells are expendable because antibodies can be replaced through periodic immunoglobulin (antibody) injections.

Surrounding tissues can be damaged by the substances that T cells make when they are fully activated. Much of the feeling of illness that occurs with an infection, including the fevers, sweats, and chills, are due to substances (called cytokines) the T cells produce to help fight the infection rather than from the infection itself. These same substances are made by the CAR T cells but at higher amounts (think T cells on steroids), producing the major side effect of CAR T cells, called cytokine release syndrome, which can occasionally be life threatening.

Bispecific antibodies are conceptually similar to CAR T cells. But instead of "arming" patients' own T cells, this approach involves manufacturing monoclonal antibodies to recognize a cancer marker, as well as a T-cell marker, enabling the T cells to better attack the cancer. Bispecific antibodies have many of the same side effects of CAR T cells but are off the shelf—they don't have to be made specially for each patient.

Bone marrow transplantation: A backhoe for dandelions

There are few examples of cancer being cured with only one modality. For all the reasons discussed earlier—vast numbers of cancer cells, their heterogeneity, and so on—curing cancer is going to require combining multiple approaches. Bone marrow transplantation has been successful as a single therapy in curing certain blood cancers and has also been effective as a combination therapy when used with other treatment types. (Although the term "stem cell transplantation" may be more commonly used and perhaps sounds sexier, Rick prefers the term "bone marrow transplantation," or BMT, because the stem cells are not the part of the transplant that cures the cancer. I'll come back to that in a bit.)

If most cancer therapies are still only lawnmowers for dandelions and other weeds in the yard, BMT can be considered a backhoe that removes both the good and bad roots, followed by resodding. This image of a backhoe digging the marrow out of your bones may be a little disturbing, so let me briefly discuss how BMT is performed. This explanation is a little heavy on science. You might find it helpful to watch Rick's 10-minute YouTube video on BMT, called "Bone Marrow Transplant: Pioneering Discovery to Curing Patients," which recently won a Telly Award.

Bone marrow is collected, or "harvested," through a needle inserted into a bone, typically the pelvic bone. Alternatively, the marrow cells can be pushed into the blood through a process called mobilization and collected through the same process used for platelet donations. These are outpatient procedures that are about as serious as going to the dentist to get one's teeth cleaned. About 2%–3% of the donor's marrow is removed (an amount so small that it would never be missed and is replaced by the body in a couple of weeks). The harvested bone marrow cells are given to the patient as a blood transfusion. At that point, the cells are able to find their way "home" to the bone marrow and are capable of regrowing new bone marrow and producing all the cells made by the bone marrow.

BMTs can take one of two forms: (1) autologous, in which the patient's own bone marrow is collected, cryopreserved (freezing the cells without killing them), and then given back, typically to replenish bone marrow after chemotherapy; or (2) allogeneic, in which bone marrow from healthy donors is used, bringing in the cavalry of a healthy immune system to join the fight. (For more information, see the Science Corners on allogeneic and autologous transplantations.) Classically, the "backhoe" portion of the procedure was the high-dose chemotherapy given immediately before the transplant, usually 5–10 times higher than standard treatment doses. It was hoped that such high-dose therapy would have a better chance of killing the cancer cells, but as a side effect it also killed normal blood cells that were also dividing fairly rapidly. The transplant, given as a blood transfusion, resods the bone marrow, rescuing the patient from the very high doses of therapy. We now know that an allogeneic transplant is a potent form of immunotherapy and acts as the backhoe removing the bad roots.

Another cool aspect of an allogeneic BMT is that the new immune system can augment the activity of new targeted therapies and immunotherapies. Combining these active, but not curing, therapies

SCIENCE CORNER

Allogeneic Transplantation

In the early days of bone marrow transplantation (BMT)—the 1970s and 80s—a transplant always used allogeneic bone marrow from a sibling who was considered a so-called perfect match. The allogeneic donor had to be a "perfect" match to prevent the transplanted immune system from perceiving the patient as foreign and attacking him or her. Called graft (transplant) versus host (patient) disease or GVHD, this reaction to the transplant could be extremely serious, resulting in life-threatening medical complications or death. Since no match is actually perfect for the purposes of BMT, the term "perfect match" meant that the patient and the transplant donor had similar immune systems and therefore there was the lowest possible risk from GVHD.

Although BMT offered cures for many patients, there were several problems with the procedure. Many patients, because of their older age or underlying medical condition, could not tolerate the very high doses of therapy that were being used to cure the cancer. Eventually it became clear that high doses of chemotherapy were not required for allogeneic transplants because the new transplanted immune system could cure the cancer.

Cancers are often invisible to the patient's own immune system, but a new immune system should be able to see the cancer as foreign and attack it. Accordingly, most allogeneic transplants no longer use high-dose therapy before the transplant; instead, they use low-dose chemotherapy and often radiation (called non-myeloablative, reduced intensity, or "mini" conditioning) to allow the newly transplanted immune system to take. Patients who receive a kidney, liver, or heart transplant require anti-rejection drugs after the transplant, usually for the rest of their lives, to prevent the body from rejecting the transplanted organ. With allogeneic BMT, the mini-conditioning given before the transplant is the anti-rejection medicine.

The lower doses of therapy made transplants tolerable to older and less fit patients, but there was still the issue of needing "perfect" matches. Thus, until recently, the holy grail of BMT was finding "perfect" donors for all the patients who desperately needed them. The recent ability to use mismatched donors for BMT has been one of

(continued)

the major advances in the field of cancer therapy. By the turn of the millennium, the development of unrelated umbilical cord blood transplants (involving blood cells from the umbilical cord of a newborn not related to the patient) allowed many patients unable to find a "perfect" match to get a mismatched transplant; the immaturity of the newborn immune system limited the toxicity of GVHD. However, the small number of cells available in the umbilical cord and the inability of the immature immune system to adequately fight infections have limited this approach.

More recently, mismatched related or haploidentical transplants, where the donor shares only one set of genes with the patient, have been shown to be safe and effective, based largely on work from Rick's group at Johns Hopkins and several other research centers around the world. First-degree relatives (parents, children, and half of siblings) are always half-matched, and 50% of second-degree relatives (grandparents, grandchildren, aunts, uncles, nieces, and nephews) are also half-matched. First cousins are half-matched 25% of the time. With a half-matched donor transplant, the risk of needing treatment for GVHD and its attendant mortality is now less than half of what it used to be with a "perfect" matched donor. This advance is due to new approaches for preventing serious GVHD. The ability to use mini-conditioning and half-matched donors now allows almost everyone in need to have a bone marrow transplant, with many transplants now done in patients up to age 80 or even older.

The extensive research that went into understanding the characteristics of successful matches that now include half-matches is described in the Science Corner "Finding the 'Perfect' Match for Allogeneic BMT."

with a new non-tolerant immune system seems to supercharge them. Most patients with what used to be the worst leukemias can now be cured by combining low-dose chemotherapy and often radiation with an allogeneic transplant followed by targeted or immune therapies.

One such example is ALL carrying the Philadelphia chromosome, mentioned previously. This leukemia was incurable in adults before allogeneic BMT was shown to cure about a third of patients. The

SCIENCE CORNER

Autologous Transplantation

Because of the limited availability of donors in the early days of allogeneic bone marrow transplantation (BMT) and the newly discovered ability to keep frozen cells alive through cryopreservation, studies of autologous transplants—using patients' own marrow to resod—started in the early 1980s. Even though cancer stem cells like to hang out in the marrow being collected and risk being reinfused into the patient with the harvests of autologous marrow cells, autologous transplants cured some patients. The relapse rate was higher than with allogeneic transplants, both because cancer stem cells were occasionally reinfused and because the new immune system might not engage in anticancer activity (as discussed in the Science Corner "Allogeneic Transplantation"). Nonetheless, autologous transplants were safer because there was no graft-versus-host disease (GVHD).

No autologous transplants were performed before 1980, but by the 1990s nearly 50,000 BMTs were performed annually worldwide, with two-thirds being autologous. Although allogeneic transplant numbers are gradually catching up to autologous numbers as the former get safer, autologous transplants still outnumber allogeneic ones. Almost all the autologous transplants now performed are for aggressive lymphomas and multiple myeloma because these diseases are sensitive to the high-dose chemotherapy that is given before the reinfusion of stem cells. Allogeneic transplants are also sometimes used in these diseases and are the usual transplants performed for patients with leukemia and myelodysplastic syndrome (MDS).

targeted therapy drug imatinib improved control of this leukemia but was unable to cure it in adults. However, when imatinib, or one of the similar newer drugs, was added after the transplant as maintenance therapy, more than 80% of patients appeared to be cured. The newly transplanted immune system can be considered a platform for enhancing the curative potential of many new agents in fighting other types of cancer.

SCIENCE CORNER

Finding the "Perfect" Match for Allogeneic BMT

When Rick started working in bone marrow transplantation (BMT), the only "perfect" matches were siblings who inherited the same two sets of genes on chromosome 6 from their two parents. These genes produce proteins called major human leukocyte (another name for white blood cell) antigens, or HLAs, which are largely responsible for controlling an individual's immune system. Donor matching was determined by HLA typing: assessing of 12 major HLA proteins or markers on white blood cells (6 inherited as a set from each parent) to see if they were the same. If the 12 markers were not the same, the risk of GVHD was so high (virtually 100%, with more than a 50% mortality rate) that a transplant was not considered safe.

It turns out there are literally hundreds of other markers, called minor HLA antigens, that influence the immune system and are not inherited as a set on chromosome 6. Thus, even "perfectly" matched siblings for major HLA proteins will likely have differences in these minor HLA antigens. Until recently, the risk of needing treatment for GVHD was about 70%, with a mortality risk of about 20%, even with a "perfect" match.

Unfortunately, there is only a 25% chance that two siblings will be "perfect" matches, so in the early days of BMT, most patients in need of BMT for curing their cancer were unable to receive this life-saving procedure. Understanding this 25% chance requires only some simple genetics and math. Two siblings have a 50% chance of getting the same gene from one parent and a 50% chance of getting the same gene from the other parent, so there is a 25% chance of getting the same two genes ($0.5 \times 0.5 = 0.25$). Because of the low likelihood of having a sibling who is a "perfect" match, worldwide banks of volunteer donors that increased the chances of finding a match started springing up in the 1990s. Unfortunately, such unrelated registries, even with the millions of potential volunteer donors currently signed up, find perfect matches for only about 50% of patients, and many ethnic groups such as African Americans and Latinos have less than a 20% chance.

I said there is no such thing as a perfect match, and you may be wondering, why isn't an identical twin the perfect match for BMT? It turns out that an identical twin is *too* perfect a match. Because the identical twins' immune systems are exact copies of one another, the transplant offers no benefit in fighting the twin's cancer. Thus, identical twins, once thought of as the perfect match for allogeneic transplants, are now rarely used for that purpose.

In summary, although most cancer patients will not need BMT, it is an example of how different types of cancer therapies can work together. Allogeneic BMT involves low doses of classic cytotoxic chemotherapy and often radiation to allow the transplant to take, or—to go back to Rick's gardening analogy—to get the soil tilled and ready for planting. The transplant brings a healthy new immune system, or immunotherapy, to the fight. Maintenance therapy is given after the transplant, adding targeted therapy to the mix to work in concert with the new immune system. Together, these different modalities are now able to cure some of what used to be the most difficult of cancers.

CHAPTER 9

Cancer Prevention I

Stop It before It Starts

DON'T SMOKE.

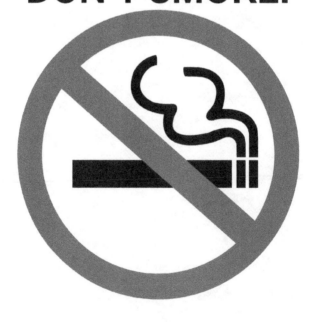

CHAPTER 10

Cancer Prevention II

Everything in Moderation (including Moderation)

THE LAST CHAPTER ON CANCER PREVENTION was short, as by far the single most important thing anyone can do to prevent cancer is to not smoke. The vast majority of environmentally related cancers, including 80%–90% of lung cancers, are the result of smoking. However, almost every aspect of life has been proposed to have an impact on cancer, though many of the data are controversial and even contradictory. It is human nature to think that most things in life, both good and bad, can be controlled, but most cancers result from normal processes of cellular self-renewal and are beyond our control.

In this chapter, I will discuss the evidence, and lack thereof, for some commonly considered strategies for preventing cancer. But I strongly suggest you consider all of these, except for the directive not to smoke, in moderation, heeding Oscar Wilde's famous quote: "Everything in moderation, including moderation." To put it another way, outside of smoking, most behaviors are likely to have at most minor effects on cancer, and the data, much of it murky, also need to be considered in moderation.

One of the major challenges in dissecting the effects of one specific behavior on cancer is that it may be impossible to separate individual behaviors that are strongly linked, even in large data sets. Individuals who smoke heavily, for example, are also prone to drink heavily and vice versa. Heavy drinkers are also often overweight. So trying to isolate the effects of alcohol on cancer is difficult because of its interaction with smoking and to a lesser extent obesity.

And no discussion on prevention would be complete without a discussion on screening for cancer, which, you may be surprised to learn, may be the most controversial part of prevention.

Put on your hip boots and get ready to wade into the depths of cancer prevention strategies and what research is telling us about the effectiveness of these strategies. Once we are done, you will understand how the National Cancer Institute came up with this graphic and why some strategies are included and some are not (figure 10.1).

Alcohol: The good, the bad, and the ugly

Perhaps no health studies are more controversial than those on alcohol. We have likely all read lots about not only the evils of alcohol but also its benefits. One study will suggest that alcohol is good in moderation, while others suggest that consuming even small amounts of alcohol is bad. We all know that heavy drinking or drinking and driving can be really ugly, damaging the liver and heart and possibly injuring or killing people. Alcohol has been associated with cancers of the mouth, throat, larynx (voice box), esophagus, stomach, liver, colon, and breast. The American Cancer Society website says: "Alcohol use accounts for about 6% of all cancers and 4% of all cancer deaths in the United States." Although the data linking alcohol and cancer

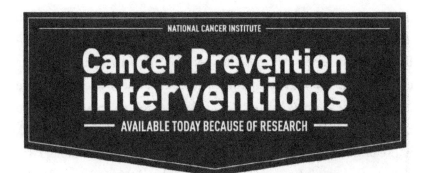

Figure 10.1. Ways to prevent cancer. (*Source:* National Cancer Institute, Division of Cancer Prevention, Cancer prevention interventions available today, 2023, https://prevention.cancer.gov/news-and-events/infographics/cancer-prevention-interventions-available-today.)

may appear bad, it might not be as ugly as it appears, in part because the associations between alcohol and cancer are complex.

Most of the data demonstrate that cancer risk is associated with the amount of alcohol someone drinks, not the type of alcoholic beverage. Unlike cigarette smoking, where many substances in tobacco smoke appear to be carcinogenic, any cancer risk related to alcohol appears to be from the alcohol itself. Exactly how alcohol causes cancer is unknown, but it likely involves several factors. Alcohol can act as an irritant, especially in the mouth, throat, and liver, where it can damage cells and produce genetic mutations, particularly in association with cigarette smoking. The metabolism of alcohol involves its conversion to acetaldehyde, a chemical that has been shown to cause cancer in lab animals by damaging DNA. Alcohol can also raise the body's levels of estrogen, which is well recognized to increase the risk of breast cancer. The official guidelines of the American Cancer Society state that it is best not to drink alcohol and that individuals who choose to drink should limit their intake to no more than two drinks a day for men and one drink a day for women.

Despite these data, there is some good news. There is experimental data that the antioxidant compound resveratrol, found in grapes used to make red wine, may have health benefits, including reducing cancer and heart disease. Multiple studies show that low to moderate alcohol consumption is associated with decreased risks of kidney cancers and lymphomas. Moreover, there is good evidence that low to moderate alcohol intake reduces the risk of developing and dying of heart disease and stroke and may reduce the risk of diabetes and dementia.

Because of the complexity of alcohol's effects on the body and its interactions with other agents (especially tobacco and genes), it is impossible to make blanket recommendations about alcohol and whether its effects on any individual will be good, bad, or ugly. It is likely that any amount of alcohol will increase your overall risk of cancer, although if you eat a healthy diet, don't smoke, and drink responsibly, that risk appears to be small. In some individuals, the positive cardiovascular effects may be higher than the negative effects on cancer risk. But if you don't drink alcohol, don't start because of potential health benefits. For many of us, Henny Youngman probably said it best: "When I read about the evils of drinking, I gave up reading."

Obesity: Weight, weight, don't tell me

Obesity has adverse effects on almost every aspect of health, increasing the risks of diabetes, hypertension, heart disease, stroke, emotional disorders, and even cancer. The body mass index (BMI) chart in figure 10.2 shows healthy and unhealthy weights for US adults based on height. A large international collaborative study led by researchers at the Harvard T.H. Chan School of Public Health and the University of Cambridge found that being overweight or obese is associated with a higher risk of dying prematurely, and the risk increases with additional pounds. To put this into real numbers, an average height man (5 feet 10 inches) earns an obesity label (BMI of 30) with a weight of 210 and an extremely obese label (BMI of 40) at 270 pounds, and an average woman (5 feet 4 inches), at 175 and 235 pounds, respectively. Men who are extremely obese have a fourfold greater risk of dying prematurely than men of normal weight.

More than a third of US adults are now classified as obese or extremely obese. The stark reality is that an extremely obese 60-year-old adult can expect a shorter life span than a non-obese similarly aged person with a slow-growing cancer such as chronic lymphocytic leukemia, low-grade lymphoma, or prostate cancer. Rick and most oncologists tell similar stories about patients they see for one of these indolent cancers who are also obese. When told their weight may be a greater health concern than their dreaded cancer, the patients often become irritated because they have come to address their cancer and not their weight.

Although many of the health issues associated with obesity are not cancer related, many are. Again, I want to stress that, like most associations between lifestyle and cancer, most of the data come from large observational studies, and such data cannot establish that any factor definitively causes cancer. Obese people may differ from their

BODY MASS INDEX (BMI) CHART

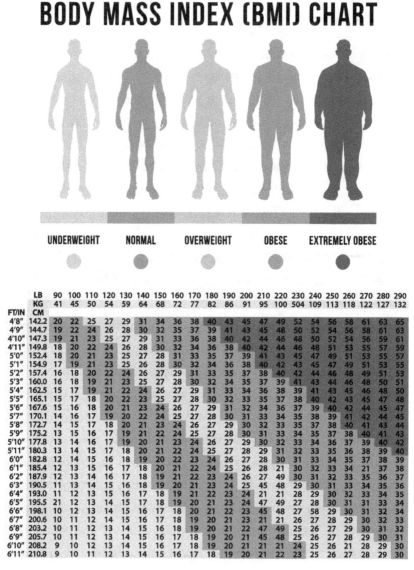

	UNDERWEIGHT	NORMAL	OVERWEIGHT	OBESE	EXTREMELY OBESE

	LB	90	100	110	120	130	140	150	160	170	180	190	200	210	220	230	240	250	260	270	280	290
	KG	41	45	50	54	59	64	68	72	77	82	86	91	95	100	504	109	113	118	122	127	132
FT/IN	CM																					
4'8"	142.2	20	22	25	27	29	31	34	36	38	40	43	45	47	49	52	54	56	58	61	63	65
4'9"	144.7	19	22	24	26	28	30	32	35	37	39	41	43	45	48	50	52	54	56	58	61	63
4'10"	147.3	19	21	23	25	27	29	31	33	36	38	40	42	44	46	48	50	52	54	56	59	61
4'11"	149.8	18	20	22	24	26	28	30	32	34	36	38	40	42	44	46	48	51	53	55	57	59
5'0"	152.4	18	20	21	23	25	27	28	31	33	35	37	39	41	43	45	47	49	51	53	55	57
5'1"	154.9	17	19	21	23	25	26	28	30	32	34	36	38	40	42	43	45	47	49	51	53	55
5'2"	157.4	16	18	20	22	24	26	27	29	31	33	35	37	38	40	42	44	46	48	49	51	53
5'3"	160.0	16	18	19	21	23	25	27	28	30	32	34	35	37	39	41	43	44	46	48	50	51
5'4"	162.5	15	17	19	21	22	24	26	27	29	31	33	34	36	38	39	41	43	45	46	48	50
5'5"	165.1	15	17	18	20	22	23	25	27	28	30	32	33	35	37	38	40	42	43	45	47	48
5'6"	167.6	15	16	18	20	21	23	24	26	27	29	31	32	34	36	37	39	40	42	44	45	47
5'7"	170.1	14	16	17	19	20	22	24	25	27	28	30	31	33	34	35	38	39	41	42	44	45
5'8"	172.7	14	15	17	18	20	21	23	24	26	27	29	30	32	33	35	37	38	40	41	43	44
5'9"	175.2	13	15	16	17	19	21	22	24	25	27	28	30	31	33	34	35	37	38	40	41	43
5'10"	177.8	13	14	16	17	19	20	21	23	24	26	27	29	30	32	33	34	36	37	39	40	42
5'11"	180.3	13	14	15	17	18	20	21	22	24	25	27	28	29	31	32	33	35	36	38	39	40
6'0"	182.8	12	14	15	16	18	19	20	22	23	24	26	27	28	30	31	33	34	35	37	38	39
6'1"	185.4	12	13	15	16	17	18	20	21	22	24	25	26	28	21	30	32	33	34	21	37	38
6'2"	187.9	12	13	14	16	17	18	19	21	22	23	24	26	27	49	30	31	32	33	35	36	37
6'3"	190.5	11	13	14	15	16	18	19	20	21	23	24	25	45	48	29	30	31	33	34	35	36
6'4"	193.0	11	12	13	15	16	17	18	19	21	22	23	24	21	28	29	30	32	33	34	35	
6'5"	195.5	21	12	13	14	15	17	18	19	20	21	23	24	47	49	27	28	30	31	31	33	34
6'6"	198.1	10	12	13	14	15	16	17	18	20	21	22	23	45	48	27	58	29	30	31	32	34
6'7"	200.6	10	11	12	14	15	16	17	18	19	20	21	23	21	21	26	27	28	29	30	32	33
6'8"	203.2	10	11	12	13	14	15	16	18	19	20	21	22	47	49	25	26	27	29	30	31	32
6'9"	205.7	10	11	12	13	14	15	16	17	18	19	20	21	45	48	25	26	27	28	29	30	31
6'10"	208.2	9	10	12	13	14	15	16	17	18	19	20	21	21	24	25	26	21	28	29	30	
6'11"	210.8	9	10	11	12	13	14	15	16	17	18	19	20	21	22	23	25	26	27	28	29	30

Figure 10.2. What's your BMI, and are you overweight?

non-obese neighbors in ways other than their weight (just as heavy drinkers also often smoke), and it is possible that their increased cancer risk may arise from factors other than obesity. With that caveat, there are significant and reliable data showing that obesity is associated with an increased risk of breast cancer, endometrial cancer, ovarian cancer, cancers of the gastrointestinal tract, and kidney cancer (figure 10.3).

Also, like alcohol, the exact ways obesity increases the risk of cancer is unclear but are likely to be multifactorial. The clearest mechanism by which obesity increases the risks of breast, endometrial, and ovarian cancer is that adipose, or fat, tissue produces excess amounts of estrogens, which are growth factors for these cancers in women. Overweight individuals are also more likely to have conditions associated with chronic inflammation, which is known to produce DNA damage that over time can cause cancer. Obesity-associated inflammations that are risk factors for certain cancers include gastroesophageal

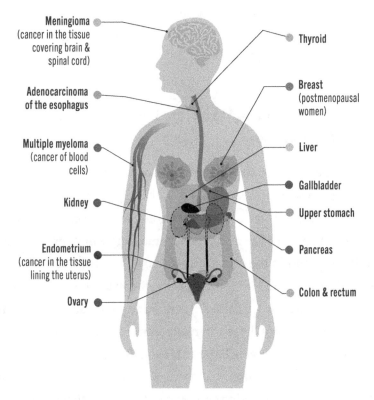

Figure 10.3. Cancers associated with overweight and obesity. (*Source:* National Cancer Institute, Cancers associated with overweight and obesity, https://www.cancer.gov/about-cancer/causes-prevention/risk/obesity/overweight-cancers-infographic.)

reflux and esophageal adenocarcinoma, gallstones and gallbladder cancer, and a form of hepatitis due to fatty liver disease.

As already discussed, there is a link between obesity and type 2 diabetes. Unlike type 1 diabetes, in which the body no longer makes insulin, type 2 diabetes is associated with normal or elevated levels of insulin due to insulin resistance induced by adipose tissue. This is why weight loss can improve or even eliminate type 2 diabetes. High levels of insulin may promote kidney, colon, and prostate cancer. Adipose tissue also makes hormones called adipokines, which may promote the growth of cancer. Finally, many studies suggest that obesity has a detrimental effect on outcomes once cancer is diagnosed. The good news is that not only can weight loss treat type 2 diabetes, but most of the increased cancer risks associated with obesity also appear to go away with weight loss.

Coffee/caffeine: If I had to choose between coffee and cancer, I'd choose . . .

The good news is that you don't have to choose between coffee and cancer (figure 10.4). Research and debates on possible links between coffee drinking and cancer have been going on for decades. Much of the concern about coffee and cancer came from a high-profile study published in 1981 in the *New England Journal of Medicine*—arguably the top clinical journal in medicine—that found a statistically significant association between drinking coffee and pancreatic cancer. This paper garnered lots of press and made intrinsic sense to many—how could anything pleasurable be good for you? Since then, however, numerous studies have found that there is in fact an inverse relationship between coffee drinking and pancreatic cancer; that is, the more coffee you drink, the lower your risk of pancreatic cancer. Recent stud-

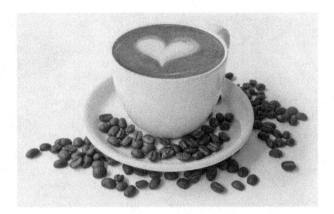

Figure 10.4. Can coffee actually be good for you? The perhaps surprising answer is an emphatic yes.

ies have shown a similar inverse relationship between coffee drinking and risk of dying from all cancers. It is critical to combine clinical findings (bedside observations) with knowledge of science (the bench), and caffeine has also shown anticancer effects in the laboratory. So how did the 1981 study get it so wrong? It turns out that any research finding has a real, though often small, possibility of coming to the wrong conclusion just by chance (see the Science Corner on probability calculations).

This means that truth can never be established by just one study or one set of experiments in the lab, regardless of how well they are run, since there is always a possibility that the outcome was the result of chance. Truth can be determined only when the data from multiple sources line up in one direction. One isolated piece of data can always be wrong. It is now clear that the data on coffee and cancer all come together so that you can comfortably follow Henry Rollins's advice: "What goes best with a cup of coffee? Another cup." The data also show that tea drinking is not a risk for cancer and if anything, like coffee, may be protective.

SCIENCE CORNER

Probability Calculations

Many of you have no doubt come across p values, commonly used to help understand statistical test results. In the simplest terms, a p value is a measure of how likely it is for a result to be due to chance. The smaller the p value, the less likely a result is due to chance or, to put it another way, the more likely the finding is real. Importantly, p values are never zero; in fact, it is common practice to say that a p value less than 0.05 (or less than 5% of the time this finding will in fact end up not being real) is "statistically significant." The operative word here is "statistically," because 5% of the time, after more studies are done, the result will be due to chance and end up not being real.

Let's dig a bit further into the role chance can play in the outcomes of experiments. As an example, let's say you want to verify that a presumably normal coin can be used for deciding who gets the football first in a sudden death playoff of a tied game. To be fair to both sides, the coin must be proven to come up heads 50% of the time. However, even if the coin is perfectly fair and balanced, heads may not come up 50% of the time, especially after a limited number of coin flips. If you flip the normal coin 10 times, 17% of the time it will come up heads 7 times, instead of 5, just by chance. (I won't go into the math here, but Rick assures me it is right.) Thus, if you were deciding whether the coin could be used for the playoff coin flip based on just 10 flips, you have a pretty good chance of determining that a normal coin appeared to be flawed.

Even if you flip the coin 20 times, heads will come up 14 times, instead of 10, 6% of the time by chance. But the more you flip a normal coin, the less likely you are to have heads come up at a frequency different from 50%: 100 flips will produce 70 heads almost never (well, 4 times in 100,000), and if you flip a normal coin 1,000 times, it will always come up heads close to 50% of the time.

The 1981 *New England Journal of Medicine* study that incorrectly suggested that coffee increased the risk of pancreatic cancer included only 1,000 participants. That may be a lot for coin flips, but it is a small sample size for complex human beings with complicated behaviors that are difficult to tease apart. For example, if coffee drinkers in 1981 were more likely than non-coffee drinkers to smoke, that would increase their pancreatic cancer risk, even if coffee initially looked like the culprit.

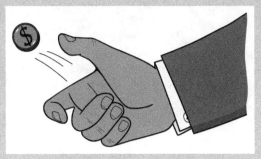

P values are just a way statisticians make coin flips seem complicated.

Ultraviolet radiation: "In a thousand years, archeologists will dig up tanning beds and think we fried people as punishment"

Other than cigarette smoking, there is no bigger preventable cause for cancer than ultraviolet radiation. Exposure to UV radiation from the sun and other sources, like tanning beds, damages DNA in skin cells that not only causes early aging of skin but also leads to cancer. Although the positives of sunlight to life on Earth certainly outweigh its negatives, the same can't be said for tanning beds (figure 10.5), as Olivia Wilde's quote introducing this section highlights.

People of all ages and skin tones should limit the amount of time they spend under UV radiation. Risks from the sun are highest between mid-morning and late afternoon, and it must be remembered that sunlight is reflected by sand, water, snow, and ice and can go through windshields and windows. Although skin cancer is more

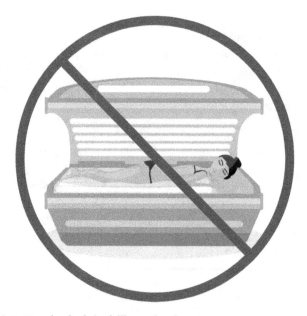

Figure 10.5. Tanning beds look like coffins for a reason.

common among lightly complected individuals, even people with dark skin can develop skin cancer. Melanin, the dark brown to black pigment that is responsible for dark skin tones, helps block out damaging UV rays up to a point. This is why people with naturally darker skin are less likely to get sunburned, but unfortunately melanin doesn't completely prevent the UV radiation–induced DNA damage to skin cells that leads to cancer.

The good news is that protecting yourself against UV radiation is quite easy. Stay out of the sun as much as you can, especially from about 10 a.m. to 4 p.m. If you work or play outside, use sunscreen that has a sun protection factor (SPF) of at least 30 and that filters both UVA and UVB rays. Use sunglasses that filter UV radiation to protect your eyes and the skin around your eyes. Wear a wide-brimmed hat, and cover your arms and legs as much as is possible and comfortable. Additionally, ultraviolet protection factor (UPF) clothing is recommended for individuals with a high skin cancer risk. Don't use tanning beds, tanning booths, or sunlamps. Regular skin checks by a doctor are important for people who have already had skin cancer or have a family history of skin cancer.

Infections: An ounce of prevention is worth a pound of cure

Most estimates suggest that infections, particularly viruses, cause about 15% of cancers worldwide but only about 7% of cancers in the United States and other high-income countries. Viral infections are the cause of most cases of cervical cancer in women, most cases of anal cancer and liver cancer, some cases of head and neck cancer, and a small number of lymphomas. Bacterial infections and even some parasites can also cause cancer. Most cancers caused by infections occur as a result of local chronic inflammation that damages DNA, as already discussed. Some viruses, however, cause cancer by directly causing cells to grow abnormally.

The hepatitis B virus (HBV) and hepatitis C virus (HCV) are the major causes of liver cancer worldwide. Both cause liver cancer by generating chronic inflammation in the liver. There are vaccines to prevent both hepatitis viruses, and both can now be treated. Bacterial infections, like *Helicobacter pylori* (*H. pylori*), the cause of stomach ulcers, can also cause stomach cancers and some lymphomas. Even some parasites, like schistosomiasis, can cause cancer. Again, cancer due to these infections is the result of chronic inflammation. *Helicobacter* and schistosomiasis can both be treated with antibiotics.

Several viruses cause cancer by directly infecting cells and causing them to grow abnormally. The three best-known examples are the Epstein-Barr virus (EBV), human papillomavirus (HPV), and the

human T-cell leukemia virus type 1 (HTLV-1). EBV causes mononucleosis as well as lymphomas and cancers of the nose and throat.
Most individuals are infected with EBV as a child or young adult,
often with just common cold symptoms, and it is never diagnosed.
EBV is a herpes virus (like the cold sore virus and chicken pox), and
like all herpes viruses remains latent in the body lifelong. Why only
rare individuals develop cancer from EBV is unknown, and there is
no treatment or vaccine.

HPV causes most cervical cancers in women as well as most anal
cancers and some cancers of the head and neck. Although there is no
treatment for HPV, it can now be prevented with a vaccine.

HTLV-1, which affects T cells, is spread by blood transfusions,
sexual contact, and needle sharing. It can also be spread from mother
to child during birth or breastfeeding. Although this virus generally
causes no signs or symptoms, some affected people may later develop adult T-cell leukemia (ATL). There is no cure or treatment for
HTLV-1, and it is considered a lifelong condition; however, 95% of
infected people remain asymptomatic their whole lives.

Ben Franklin's famous quote "an ounce of prevention is worth a
pound of cure" is perhaps most relevant in relation to infections causing cancer, since they can usually be prevented by immunization or
treatment of the infection.

Diet: You are what you eat

Rick gets more questions about diet as a treatment or prevention for
cancer than about any other single topic. One of the reasons for this
is undoubtedly that our moms drilled into us—correctly—how important a good diet is. We've learned that we are what we eat.

As we know, it is human nature to believe there are causes for untoward events that we can influence by modifying our environment.

Studies into the effects of diet on cancer have been going on for decades. The hope is that some component of the diet is associated with a higher or lower risk of cancer. Some laboratory studies have even suggested that certain dietary compounds may cause or prevent cancer. Just about every known vitamin has been claimed to prevent or treat cancer, as have a raft of herbal supplements and alternative and "miracle-cure" diets.

Let's discuss some specifics about diet and cancer. Chemicals present in charred red meat can cause cancers in laboratory animals, and although some studies in humans have suggested an association, others have not. In the laboratory, antioxidants such as vitamin E block the activity of other chemicals, known as free radicals, that may damage DNA in cells, but research in humans has not convincingly demonstrated a protective effect against cancer. Some laboratory studies have even suggested that antioxidants may promote cancer. Concerns about artificial sweeteners and cancer arose when very high doses of saccharin were found to cause bladder cancer in laboratory animals. However, saccharin and newer artificial sweeteners have never been shown to cause cancer in humans. Several substances in cruciferous vegetables (cabbage family), such as cabbage itself, broccoli, cauliflower, Brussels sprouts, and kale, have long been touted for their health benefits, including cancer prevention. Although cruciferous vegetables are excellent sources of many vitamins and minerals as well as fiber, all of which can promote health, there is no clear evidence that these vegetables have anticancer properties.

Finally, the number of special diets for cancer is too numerous to discuss in depth, but let's talk about a few of the most publicized. Macrobiotic diets are the ones discussed the most by Rick's patients. Although there is no one macrobiotic diet, these diets typically avoid meat and poultry, animal fats (such as lard and butter), eggs, dairy products, refined sugar, and foods containing artificial sweeteners or other chemical additives. Recommended foods are preferably organically grown and minimally processed. Consumption of genetically modified foods is also discouraged. Although there are aspects of macrobiotic diets that may promote health, there is no evidence that they have any anticancer properties. Moreover, macrobiotic diets may be deficient in vitamins B_{12} and D, as well as calcium.

Another highly touted anticancer diet is the Gerson diet, which is based on the premise that the body's immune system can be enhanced to cure disease by removing toxins from the body and replacing excess salt in the body's cells with potassium. The Gerson diet has three basic components: a strict organic vegetarian diet made up of fruits and vegetables high in potassium and low in sodium; vitamin, mineral, and enzyme supplements; and coffee or castor oil enemas. Not only has scientific research found no evidence that the Gerson diet stimulates anticancer activity, but it also may not be the best diet for patients to follow when they are ill and already undernourished. In addition, frequent enemas can be harmful.

Another diet supposed to have anticancer activity is the ketogenic, or keto, diet, which consists of foods that are high in fat, moderate to low in protein, and very low in carbohydrates. The concept is to "starve" cancer cells by preventing the cells from using glucose for energy and growth. As with other so-called anticancer diets, there is no good evidence that a keto diet benefits cancer patients. Moreover, such a diet may cause kidney damage, higher cholesterol levels, unintentional weight and bone loss, and certain vitamin and mineral deficiencies.

In summary, no diet or food has been proven to cause or cure cancer. The motto "everything in moderation" is important when it comes to both individual food items and your diet in general. Now that super-sized portions are a staple of the American diet, it is all too easy to eat to excess. When Rick's patients ask what foods to eat or avoid, his usual response is to recommend a normal, well-rounded, balanced diet, just like your mother recommended. Nothing more, nothing less. And if you are eating your mother's cooking, clean your plate; otherwise, set aside some of your restaurant meal for a later snack.

Environmental risk factors: "Unable to attribute misfortune to chance . . . the people looked for monsters in their midst"

Exposure to chemicals and other substances in the environment has been linked to some cancers. The list of toxins that can cause cancer (carcinogens) is endless, and we've all heard about environmental cancer outbreaks like those that occurred at Love Canal in the 1970s. Although many toxins cause cancer in laboratory animals (and perhaps in humans who are exposed to large quantities of those toxins), they are unlikely to be involved in the development of cancer in more than a few isolated patients. Air pollution, power lines, hair dyes, pesticides, and other pollutants are all believed to cause cancer. Drinking water that contains a large amount of arsenic has been linked to skin, bladder, and lung cancers. Linking carcinogens to cancer in humans in scientific studies, however, has been particularly challenging because of the need to control confounding variables over prolonged periods of time.

Love Canal, near Buffalo, New York, is a prime example of the difficulty of attributing cancer risk to environmental toxins. Near the end of the nineteenth century, William T. Love began excavating a canal that would bypass Niagara Falls on the Niagara River, allowing boats to travel between Lake Erie and Lake Ontario. The diverted water was to be used to generate hydroelectric power. With a seemingly limitless supply of energy, he imagined that new industries would spring up and produce an economic boom for the area. Love also envisioned a planned community, which he would call Model City, where workers flocking to the area would live.

After digging less than a mile of his canal, Love went bankrupt, in part because of the introduction of alternating current generators and transformers that allowed electricity to be produced and transported across the country. In the 1920s his fallow Love Canal became a dump site for municipal waste from the city of Niagara Falls, and in the 1940s it was purchased by Hooker Chemical Company, now Occidental Chemical Corporation, for the same purpose. Ultimately, nearly 20,000 tons of chemical waste, including benzene and dioxin from the manufacture of dyes, perfumes, and rubber, were deposited in the site. In 1953 the dump, then closed and covered with dirt, was given for a token payment of $1 to the local school board with a liability limitation clause that released the company from all legal obligations should lawsuits later occur.

Despite the understanding that the land was filled with chemical waste, an elementary school was built there. The school opened in 1955, and that same year, a large area in the schoolyard crumbled, exposing drums for toxic chemicals, which filled with water during rainstorms. Children enjoyed playing in the large puddles that were created. Land bordering the canal was also sold and developed, and by the 1970s residents were complaining about strange odors and substances in their yards. When an official from the Environmental Protection Agency came to inspect the area, he saw rusting barrels of waste that had worked their way above ground. Waste oozed into several backyards and seeped into the basement of at least one home. Laboratory analyses of soil samples showed the presence of more than 200 distinct organic chemical compounds, many of which were considered toxins.

By 1978, Love Canal had become a national media story with articles referring to the neighborhood as "a public health time bomb." In the summer of 1978, President Jimmy Carter proclaimed Love Canal a federal health emergency and ordered the Federal Disaster Assistance Administration to help the city of Niagara Falls with cleanup. Two years later, Congress passed the Superfund Act to clean up hazardous waste sites, with the Love Canal the first beneficiary.

So, how many cancers were related to the Love Canal? Initially, the EPA estimated that people living along the Love Canal stood a 1 in 10 chance of getting cancer during their lives. But soon thereafter, the agency admitted to a mathematical error; the increased risk was in fact 1 in 100, which was less than the rest of the state of New York. The lack of increased mortality in Love Canal residents was later confirmed by a New York state study with 20 years of follow-up (figure 10.6). There is no question that Love Canal is an unfortunate story, and some individuals certainly suffered health consequences. For example, the birth defect rate for children born near the canal was higher than in the rest of the state. However, the conclusion that this tragedy produced no increased cancers underscores not only the rarity of cancers caused by specific environmental toxins but also the difficulty proving causation.

As I've already discussed, there is an innate human need to ascribe a cause to calamitous events rather than just accepting that some bad outcomes are a result of bad luck. This is highlighted in one of Rick's favorite quotes from Bernard Beckett's book *Genesis*: "Unable to attribute misfortune to chance, unable to accept their ultimate insignificance within the greater scheme, the people looked for monsters in their midst."

Despite the lack of evidence for cancer causation by most environmental toxins such as hair dyes, power lines, and pesticides, there truly are some notable "monsters in our midst." The association

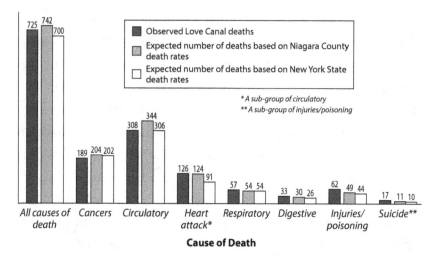

Figure 10.6. Observed versus "expected" deaths in Love Canal, 1979–1996. Initial reports of higher-than-expected cases of cancer around Love Canal were in reality the result of a mathematical error. In actuality, the incidence was the same as the rest of the state. (*Source:* New York State Department of Health, *Love Canal follow-up health study: mortality community report*, published July 2008, revised May 2017, https://www.health.ny.gov/environmental/investigations/love_canal/mortality_community_report.htm.)

between asbestos and cancer, especially mesothelioma, a form of cancer that involves the thin lining of the chest and abdominal cavities, is clear. Asbestos exposure is especially problematic in smokers. Asbestos is the name given to a group of fibrous materials that occur naturally in the environment, do not conduct electricity, and are resistant to heat, fire, and chemicals. For these reasons, asbestos was widely used for insulation and fireproofing in homes and ships, as well as in an almost endless variety of other products such as automotive brakes.

If products containing asbestos are disturbed, as they might be during repairs, tiny asbestos fibers are released into the air. The fibers can get trapped in the lungs of anyone who breathes them in and remain there essentially forever. Over time, accumulated asbestos fibers can cause chronic inflammation and scarring, which can affect breathing as well as lead to cancer (there's that link between inflammation and cancer again). Based on the overwhelming evidence of asbestos's ill effects on health, the United States banned the use of asbestos, initially in gas fireplaces, and by 1989 for all new uses.

Another monster in our midst is radon, an invisible, odorless radioactive gas that, outside of smoking, is the major cause of lung cancer. Radon, which is released from the normal decay of radioactive substances in rocks and soil, seeps up from the ground and diffuses into the air. It is usually present at very low levels outdoors, and everyone breathes in tiny quantities of it every day. In areas without adequate ventilation, however, such as poorly ventilated underground rooms in homes and other buildings, radon can accumulate to levels that substantially increase the risk of lung cancer. Testing is the only way to know if a home or building has elevated radon levels, and most commercially available radon detectors do an excellent job (if plugged in and the battery is working).

Yet another monster is benzene, a real, but rare, cause of leukemia. Benzene is a colorless, flammable liquid with a sweet odor that evaporates quickly when exposed to air. It is among the 20 most widely used chemicals in the United States, primarily as a starting material in making other chemicals. It is also found in cigarette smoke, which accounts for about half of US benzene exposure.

Screening for cancer: Early diagnosis or overdiagnosis

Screening for cancer means looking for warning signs of cancer before it causes any signs or symptoms. Intuitively, screening seems like an obvious and important approach to preventing the complications of cancer, but it is actually quite controversial. Although the terms "early detection" and "screening" are often used interchangeably, they are not quite the same. In a literal sense, a screen prevents pests from getting in—as a screen door keeps insects out—while early detection involves hunting out pests that do get in before they can multiply and cause problems. Is there such a thing as screening that can prevent cancer from getting in the body? The answer is yes—detecting and removing precancerous lesions before they become cancer is the prime example of successful cancer screening. This is the concept behind Pap tests, procedures to look for colon polyps, and skin examinations for atypical moles, all of which attempt to prevent precancerous lesions from becoming actual cancer.

In contrast, many so-called cancer screening procedures, including PSA for prostate cancer and mammography for breast cancer, would more accurately be called early detection strategies. These approaches try to detect cancer while it is still localized so that removing it can prevent it from spreading. Early detection strategies such as PSA screening and mammography have recently become quite controversial.

Let's start with true cancer screening, or the detection of precancerous lesions so that they can be removed before developing into cancer. Perhaps the most successful of all cancer screening procedures is cervical cancer screening, an essential part of a woman's routine health care. Routine screening for cervical cancer significantly reduces the development of, and deaths from, cervical cancer. Nearly all cases of cervical cancer are caused by infection with sexually transmitted HPV virus.

Cervical cancer screening is done by scraping cells from the cervix; the scrapings are sent to a laboratory, where they are examined under a microscope for abnormal-looking cells (the Pap smear or test) and/or tested for the presence of HPV. Women ages 21 through 29 should be screened with a Pap test every three years, and women ages 30 through 65 should be screened every five years with Pap and HPV testing or every three years with a Pap test alone. These screening intervals were established to balance false positives (test results that report you have a specific condition when you don't) and false negatives (test results that report you don't have a specific condition when in fact you do). Most HPV infections are controlled by the immune system over the course of one to two years. Thus, testing too frequently would result in false positives. At the same time, it is important to limit the possibility of false negatives—that is, missed illness—by testing frequently enough so as not to delay the diagnosis and treatment of a precancerous condition.

Screening for precancerous colon polyps is highly successful in preventing colon cancer, the third most common cancer. However, whereas more than 80% of women have cervical cancer screening, less than two-thirds of adults undergo colon cancer screening. Historically, effective colon cancer screening required routine colonoscopy, but more recently virtual colonoscopy and stool DNA tests have also been shown to be useful.

A colonoscopy involves examining the entire length of the colon (or large intestine) using a thin, tubelike instrument with a light and a lens for viewing, along with a tool for removing polyps. This procedure sounds worse than it is. Light anesthesia makes it pain free, and there are few risks, which are mostly limited to adverse reactions to the anesthetic or bleeding if a tissue sample, or biopsy, is taken. And of course, there is still the "inconvenient" day of prep.

A virtual colonoscopy entails using a CT scanner to produce a series of pictures of the colon from outside the body. This eliminates the "instrument" and any associated risks but still requires the prep, as well as an actual colonoscopy if polyps are found. DNA stool tests, the easiest screening procedure for polyps, are quite sensitive but can be abnormal in the absence of polyps (in other words, false positives). Moreover, as with a virtual colonoscopy, an actual colonos-copy is required if the test is positive. Virtual colonoscopies and stool DNA tests are thus most useful for individuals at average risk for co-lon cancer who previously had a negative colonoscopy.

Although recommendations differ slightly, most groups recom-mend that individuals at average risk get screened at age 50 until age 75. If the first screen is negative, intervals of 10 years are probably sufficient, but if polyps are found, intervals of 5 years are recom-mended. These screening intervals are based on the slow natural history of the development of colon polyps and cancer. Screening should start at an earlier age in those with a family history of colon polyps or cancer.

Let's move on to a more controversial target of early detection and one that is of particular interest to Rick, myself, and all men over a cer-tain age. Prostate cancer is the most common non-skin cancer, and the second leading cause of cancer deaths, among men in the United States. There may be no more hotly debated area in cancer currently than PSA screening for prostate cancer. PSA, or prostate-specific an-tigen, is a protein secreted into the blood by normal, as well as can-cerous, prostate cells. PSA levels in the blood are usually elevated in men with prostate cancer, and the PSA test was originally approved by the Food and Drug Administration in the late 1980s to monitor the behavior of prostate cancer in men already diagnosed with the dis-ease. In 1994 the FDA additionally approved PSA in conjunction with a digital rectal exam to screen asymptomatic men for prostate cancer. Although a PSA of 4 was once considered the cutoff between normal and abnormal, there is now no clear consensus regarding the optimal PSA threshold for recommending a prostate biopsy. In general, however, the higher the PSA level, the more likely prostate cancer will be found. A continuous rise in PSA levels over time is also concerning.

That normal prostate cells also secrete PSA leads to one of the major problems already mentioned with all screening procedures: false positives. The benign conditions that elevate PSA are prostatitis (inflammation of the prostate) and benign prostatic hyperplasia (BPH, or enlargement of the prostate). As they age, most men will eventually develop BPH, so most men with elevated PSA levels turn out not to have prostate cancer on a prostate biopsy. Not surprisingly, false-positive screening tests for cancer of any variety cause anxiety and are usually followed by additional tests and procedures, like a biopsy that potentially can cause harm.

By the turn of this millennium, it had become standard practice to recommend annual PSA screening for prostate cancer in men over age 50, and even in younger men, such as African Americans, at high risk for prostate cancer. Although Medicare and many private insurers still cover annual PSA screening in men over 50, many groups and doctors no longer recommend it. Moreover, most cancer organizations no longer make specific recommendations about PSA screening and just suggest that men discuss the pros and cons with their doctors. The main pro is that PSA screening can help detect small-sized cancers before they cause symptoms.

There are lots of cons, in addition to the risks and anxiety of false positives. Finding a small cancer may not necessarily reduce a man's chance of dying from prostate cancer, since many small-sized cancers found through PSA testing grow so slowly that they are unlikely to ever threaten his life. Detecting cancers that may never become life threatening is called "overdiagnosis," and treating these cancers is called "overtreatment." Overtreatment exposes men unnecessarily to the potential complications and harmful side effects of surgery and radiation therapy, including urinary incontinence (inability to control urine flow), problems with bowel function, erectile dysfunction (loss of erections, or having erections that are inadequate for sexual intercourse), and infections. In addition, as already discussed, finding cancer "early" is really a misnomer and will not help men who have aggressive cancers that have already spread to other parts of the body.

Several randomized trials of PSA screening for prostate cancer have been carried out. All show that more cancers are detected in screened individuals, but their findings conflict on whether screening lessens mortality from prostate cancer. The US Preventive Services Task Force has developed a consensus statement after analyzing the data from all reported prostate cancer screening trials. This group estimates that for every 1,000 men ages 55 to 69 who are screened regularly, about 1 death from prostate cancer would be avoided. To save this one life per 1,000,

- 120 men would have false-positive tests that result in biopsies producing moderately bothersome symptoms in some of them;
- 100 men would be diagnosed with prostate cancer;
- of those 100 men, 80 would be treated with surgery or radiation; and
- at least 60 of these men would have a serious complication from treatment, such as erectile dysfunction and/or urinary incontinence.

Are all these biopsies and treatments necessary? You can see why PSA screening is such a contentious topic and why major organizations dealing with cancer are unwilling to give firm recommendations. When I asked Rick what he advises regarding PSA screening, he also declined to make a recommendation, saying that he was a simple blood cancer doctor. I'm 70 and have been taking PSA tests for 15 years. A few times they have been above 4 but have always gone back down. If I get another test and it is positive, I'll just wait for the next test. So I often wonder, why bother? At this point, odds are good that even if I die *with* prostate cancer, I won't die *because* of it. Perhaps screening 1,000 men to avoid one cancer death may not be worth the cost and the associated complications.

A variety of other blood tests initially developed to follow cancer that had already been diagnosed have been proposed for cancer screening. These include alpha-fetoprotein for liver cancer, CA-125 for ovarian cancer, and new DNA tests (also known as liquid biopsies) for a variety of different cancers. In general, they have not been found to effectively screen for cancer, largely because of issues similar to those just discussed with PSA screening. However, as these tests become more powerful, their utility should improve.

Lung cancer is the most common cancer, and the leading cause of death from cancer, in both men and women. It accounts for almost a quarter of all cancer deaths in the United States. The vast majority—nearly 80%—of lung cancers have spread by the time of diagnosis and are associated with poor survivals. However, several studies have found a benefit for annual lung cancer screening with low-dose CT scans in some adults: those who are over 55 years in relatively good health, currently smoke or have quit within the past 15 years, and have at least a 30 pack-year smoking history (that is, 1 pack a day for 30 years or 2 packs a day for 15 years or 3 packs a day for 10 years).

Finally, let's discuss one last early detection procedure that is becoming almost as controversial as PSA screening: screening mammography for breast cancer. A mammogram is an x-ray picture of the breast that can be used either to detect lumps that can't be felt or to check for breast cancer after a lump or other sign or symptom appears. This latter type of mammogram, called a diagnostic mammogram, is not at all controversial. According to the American Cancer Society, death rates from breast cancer have been falling since the 1980s, an outcome that is at least partly attributed to earlier detection as a result of breast cancer screening. This has led most groups involved with breast cancer to recommend that all women undergo mammograms yearly starting by age 45 and every other year beginning at age 55.

However, recent studies have questioned whether mammograms truly decrease mortality related to breast cancer. The largest study of screening mammograms was published in *JAMA Internal Medicine* in 2015. It found that screening mammograms led to a 16% increase in breast cancer diagnosis but no reduction in breast cancer deaths. Several other studies have confirmed these findings, including a study published in the *Annals of Internal Medicine* in 2017 that included all women diagnosed with invasive breast cancer in Denmark between 1980 and 2010.

These studies bring up the same discussion points I talked about with PSA in prostate cancer: screening mammograms lead to overdiagnosis with a substantial increase in the diagnosis of non-advanced cancers but no reduction in the incidence of advanced cancer. Here too, such overdiagnosis leads to overtreatment, including surgery, radiation, and adjuvant chemotherapy.

Another important concept brought up by these studies is lead-time bias, which complicates analysis of all early detection studies. Survival for patients with cancer is usually measured from the day they are diagnosed until the day they die. If a screening test leads to a diagnosis before a patient has any symptoms, the patient's survival time is increased simply because the date of diagnosis is earlier than it would have been if the diagnosis had been made when the patient had symptoms. This increase in survival time makes it seem as though screened patients are living longer when that may not be happening. It could be that the only reason survival appears longer is that the date of diagnosis is earlier for the screened patients, while the screened patients may die at the same time (from dormant metastatic disease, as discussed in chapter 4) as they would have without the screening test. Lead-time bias is really just a different way of saying that because most of the cancer's history has occurred by the time it is diagnosed, metastases are likely to have already occurred. Despite the controversy, most groups involved in breast cancer still recommend regular mammograms, although recommendations about the age to start and the frequency have generally been liberalized a bit.

Prophylactic mastectomy: The Angelina Jolie effect

Perhaps the most extreme example of prevention is the decision by some individuals to eliminate cancer risk completely through surgery so that screening is unnecessary. A so-called preventive or risk-reducing mastectomy is the surgical removal of one or both breasts in order to prevent or reduce the risk of breast cancer in women at high risk. The procedure involves either a total mastectomy (including the nipple) or removal of only the breast tissue, with the nipple left intact. A total mastectomy is usually recommended because it removes more tissue and provides the greatest protection against the development of cancer in any remaining breast tissue.

Removing both breasts is most often considered in women who have an inherited genetic mutation (*BRCA1* or *BRCA2*) associated with an elevated risk of breast cancer or who have a strong family history of breast cancer. More and more women are choosing this option, which gained public attention in 2013, when the actress Angelina Jolie underwent the procedure for her *BRCA1* mutation. In other cases, women who have had cancer in one breast may decide to have the other breast removed. Women with inherited *BRCA1* or *BRCA2* mutations are also at elevated risk for developing ovarian cancer and may decide to have prophylactic oophorectomies, or removal of the ovaries. Other women may choose prophylactic oophorectomies over prophylactic mastectomies since they reduce the risk of both ovarian and breast cancer, although they are not quite as effective in preventing breast cancer as prophylactic mastectomies.

Summary: The wisdom of Oscar Wilde and Olivia Wilde

"Everything in moderation, including moderation" does *not* mean

- enjoy a few cigarettes;
- drink all the wine, beer, and liquor you want, but avoid heavy drinking;
- forget about weight gain if you are eating good food like a 22-ounce steak;
- go to tanning salons only in preparation for spring break;
- move into an old house with radon and asbestos as long as you take some long vacations; or
- immediately schedule a whole-body scan or screening.

What we *do* mean by "everything in moderation" is: be sensible. At one extreme, don't throw in the towel in despair, believing that cancer is inevitable so it's no use doing anything. At the other extreme, don't go crazy following the latest "big thing"—the Internet's version of snake oil peddlers selling elixirs that "cure" all ailments. Pay attention to what your doctor recommends, and use the wealth of information available on reputable sites like the National Cancer Institute's web page (see Online Resources at the end of this book). Be a smart card player and enjoy the game.

CHAPTER 11

How I Learned to Stop Worrying and Not Fear Cancer

I STARTED THE BOOK POINTING OUT that "How I learned to stop worrying and not fear cancer" was a tribute to one of Rick's favorite movies, *Dr. Strangelove or: How I Learned to Stop Worrying and Love the Bomb* (figure 11.1). Why did we jointly choose this dark comedy movie reference for the last chapter of this book about cancer's myths and mysteries?

When Rick and I were growing up, it's fair to say that the biggest worry for many of us was the Cold War and its major threat, "the bomb." By exaggerating the threat of nuclear war to the extreme—I won't spoil the ending for those who haven't seen it—*Dr. Strangelove* is both funny and "disarming." Alright, maybe no one ends up *loving* the bomb other than Slim Pickens, who plays Major T. J. "King" Kong. But when compared with the movie's crazy extremes, the real-world politics at the time seemed tame and perhaps less scary. In contrast, our goal for this book was to present what is known and not known

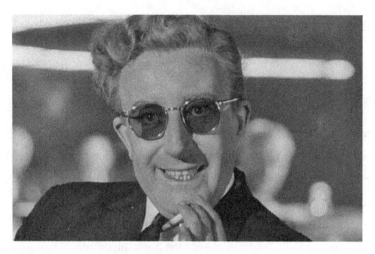

Figure 11.1. Dr. Strangelove, not worrying about the bomb or cancer.

about cancer—the facts—without exaggeration and to interject humor to lighten what can be a dark topic.

Rick is convinced that keeping a sense of humor about cancer is essential, and hopefully that has come through in this book. Laughter, after all, is often the best medicine. We hope that the chapter title helps make the point that despite its often bleak outlook and life-threatening (and definitely life-altering) consequences, every day there is more hope for patients with cancer. Not only can almost everyone with a cancer diagnosis expect to survive much longer than was possible just a quarter of a century ago but, most important, more than half will be cured. Moreover, advances in cancer treatments are coming fast and furious, so these outcomes are only going to improve, perhaps exponentially. These therapeutic advancements are particularly critical, as cancer is never going to go away. Just the opposite. At least 40% of us will develop cancer sometime in our lives, and this percentage is likely to increase as we live longer, healthier lives. All of us will certainly be impacted by the disease when it affects friends and relatives.

Cancer and aging: Live long and prosper

Despite the human need to find modifiable causes for all things that happen to us, it is clear that luck—good and bad—plays a big part in our lives. There certainly are some modifiable behaviors that can limit the risk of getting cancer—notably, not smoking (drop that cigarette, Dr. Strangelove), checking for radon, and vaccinating against certain viruses—but most cancers turn out to be merely consequences of being human. Making new cells to replace the old ones, or cell division, is not a perfect process and occasionally produces mistakes during the copying of genes.

As we live healthier lives, enabling most of us to live into our 80s and beyond, genetic mistakes will more than likely get past the immune system, the body's built-in cancer surveillance mechanism. But as discussed throughout the book, cancer must evolve through multiple mutations, which takes time. Although the lifetime risk of cancer is about 40%, 60% of people diagnosed with cancer are over 65 years of age, making cancer seem like an epidemic in older individuals. Thus, if we can avoid dying of another cause and live long enough—as is thankfully happening more and more—we will likely have cancer, even if it is never diagnosed. When and if this happens is in most cases the luck—good or bad—of the draw.

If we want to follow Mr. Spock's advice and "live long and prosper" (figure 11.2), then leading a healthy lifestyle and avoiding certain cancer triggers, such as smoking and obesity, are great steps in the right direction. Many of us keep telling ourselves 70 is the new 40, but there is science to back up that statement. A recent study found that individuals in their 70s who have been exercising regularly for

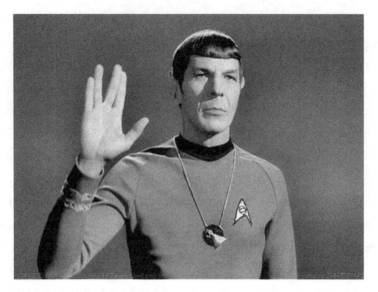

Figure 11.2. "Live long and prosper."

decades are about as strong and have the heart and lung capacities of healthy people in their 40s. Hopefully this book has provided a practical map of the cancer universe so that you can "boldly go" where you have not gone before.

"I never take too much credit when things go well, nor accept too much blame when they don't"

Rick tells me that more than half of his patients can now expect to survive longer than five years (the old definition of cure, which we now know is overly simplistic). He will not let me pin him down on an exact percentage because, as mentioned earlier, survival rates across a population aren't prescriptive for an individual and can be misleading if taken too literally. It turns out that not just most of Rick's patients but most patients with all types of cancer can now expect to survive for five years, regardless of their doctor.

So what determines whose cancer is cured, whose is not, and how long a cancer patient will survive? Is it a patient's constitution, positive or negative attitude, or intensity of prayer? There is absolutely no evidence that attitude, strength of character, or prayer plays a role in outcomes of cancer treatment. How about the love and support of friends and family? For sure, a nurturing support structure will enhance the cancer journey, but there is no data to show that it influences a longer life with cancer or a cure.

The simple answer to what determines the long-term survival of a cancer patient is the biology of the cancer itself, and some luck. Before treatment even starts, cancer, consisting of around a trillion cells at diagnosis, is already programmed to be cured or not cured, based on all of the biologic factors already discussed. Cancer researchers and clinicians are learning more every day about what those factors are, and they are using this knowledge to improve treatments and to extend life with cancer. At this time, many of these factors cannot yet be determined or addressed, but researchers are working to extend this knowledge as part of personalized, or precision, medicine. With precision medicine everyone will not get the same therapy; rather, new therapies specific to each patient's individual cancer will offer a chance of cure to people whose cancers were previously considered incurable.

At the five-year mark after cancer treatment—an arbitrary point in time and one that is too early to assess cure for many low-grade/ slow-growing cancers—patients often profusely thank their doctor for curing them. Rick has a standard response to this gratitude: "I appreciate the kind words, but I never take too much credit when things go well nor accept too much blame when they don't, because much of the outcome is out of my hands." Conversely, many patients and families blame themselves or their doctor when the cancer is not controlled. Many of us have no doubt heard patients and families lament that they would have done better if they had just fought harder, prayed more, or chosen a different doctor or treatment. Rick tell patients that the outcome is out of his hands, the patients' hands, and their families' hands even before patients start treatment.

Second opinions: Shop for the best deal, but buyer beware

Most of the time, patients do not choose the oncologist they first see. Patients, while still getting over the shock of the diagnosis, usually follow the recommendation for cancer care provided by the non-oncology provider who made the cancer diagnosis. The good news is that the outcome of cancer therapy is usually not dependent on some special expertise of the doctor. That is not to say, however, that patients should not seek second opinions. There have been 100 new anticancer agents approved since the turn of the millennium, including 30 in just 2018 and 2019. Many are used exclusively or primarily in one cancer type, and some have completely changed the treatment paradigm for a specific cancer. So how can any oncologist keep up with this ever-changing landscape? The answer is that one single oncologist can't. More and more oncologists are subspecializing in certain cancers in order to keep up. Rick used to treat all blood cancers, but now limits his practice to lymphomas and bone marrow transplantation because of the difficulty of keeping up with all the new therapies for the different cancers.

Ultimately, it is the patient's choice, not the oncologist's, whether to seek a second opinion. And there is no reason to feel embarrassed if you want one or two other opinions. How do you know if you need a second opinion? As mentioned, your oncologist can help you to know whether your cancer is straightforward and common or complex and unusual and, if asked, can likely offer suggestions for a second opinion. In general, first and second opinions will usually align, and it can be reassuring for a patient to have the first opinion reinforced. But how do you know what to do if the opinions don't align? Some detective work on your own using reputable cancer websites can be of enormous help. The approach to many cancers is straightforward. Diagnostic results are clear and sufficient to establish the best treatment plan, which might be simply watchful waiting and monitoring. The approach to other cancers can be complex or is in rapid evolution. In these complex cases, your local oncologist will likely recommend a second opinion with a cancer subspecialist.

The good news is that most patients will not have to travel great distances to the best-known cancer centers like the Mayo Clinic, Johns Hopkins, Dana-Farber, Sloan Kettering, or MD Anderson to get the most up-to-date recommendations. Virtually all medical schools have a reputable expert in all specific cancer types. You can rest assured that all such experts are networked into the best—which may or may not be the newest—treatments available.

On rare occasions, a patient may have to travel to a cancer center that offers a promising new experimental approach. In the early part of this millennium, Rick's group at Johns Hopkins was developing mismatched allogeneic transplants. Although the procedure is now the standard of care around the world, at that time they were the only ones performing the procedure in a clinical trial, and patients who could not find a match in registries needed to travel to Baltimore for that life-saving treatment.

In the following paragraphs, we offer several suggestions when seeking second opinions. First, let us caution against too many "second" opinions (figure 11.3). It is only natural for patients to "shop" for the best deal. Since an expert in a particular cancer type will generally know about promising studies at other institutions, it is unlikely that such shopping will turn up promising new therapies that experts

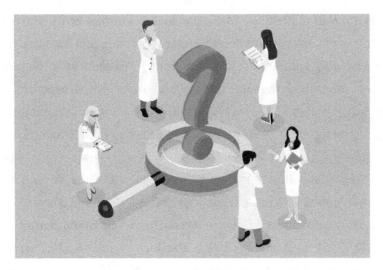

Figure 11.3. A warning about too many "second opinions": a second opinion might be important or even critical, but be cautious.

outside the institution offering the new therapy are not aware of. A patient may also try to look for the best outcomes among similar treatments, but this is definitely an area where the term "buyer beware" applies.

Interpreting treatment outcomes

It is common for patients to ask doctors to give them the outcomes they have had with a specific cancer, or occasionally some doctors will flaunt their outstanding results. Comparing results between doctors or centers is a critical area where "buyer beware" applies. To better understand how to interpret reported treatment outcomes, we need to return to our discussion of p values and the coin flip analogy. An understanding of simple statistics tells us that, depending on the number of coin flips, even a perfectly balanced coin often will not come up heads half of the time. The same general concept holds true for a doctor's or institution's cancer treatment outcomes. Let's assume that one year 100 different doctors each treat 50 patients with the same type of cancer with the same therapy, and the overall cure rate among the 5,000 patients is 70%. The actual cure rate seen in the individual doctors' groups of 50 patients will range from 57% to 83%, just by chance, like the coin flips.

Now, if the 100 doctors each treat only 10 patients with this therapy—probably a more realistic scenario for a single disease—the cure rates actually seen in those 10 patient groups would range from 33% to 100%, again just by chance. The doctors with a 100% cure rate appear to be better doctors than the ones with a 33% cure rate, when in actuality their outcomes are the same, except for statistical chance.

When shopping for the best deal, a patient should ask the doctor not what that specific doctor's outcomes have been, but what the expected chance of cure would be based on 1,000 or 5,000 patients. Using this yardstick, all 100 doctors should answer that the cure rate is 70%.

A further complication when comparing cure rates between doctors is that patient outcomes depend on many factors other than just the type of cancer. One center may have treated older patients or patients with more advanced disease, both known adverse risk factors for outcomes. It is well recognized that outcomes of new treatments are inevitably better in initial clinical trials, which typically exclude older and sicker patients as researchers seek to make sure the treatment is safe. In subsequent trials, even with the same doctors at the same institution, the results are usually not as good because once the approach has been shown to be safe, older and sicker patients are accepted for treatment.

Doctors will often point out differences in how they implement a particular treatment compared with other doctors. These differences can involve chemotherapy doses or timing, choices about inpatient or outpatient treatment, or the use of ancillary measures like antiemetics (medications that limit nausea and vomiting) or antibiotics. This is particularly true in bone marrow transplantation (BMT), where there are many moving parts that can be modified. As the director of the BMT Program at Johns Hopkins, Rick sees quite a few patients shopping for the best BMT "deal." When a patient asks who has the best deal, his standard answer is to tell them about his favorite hors d'oeuvre, guacamole. I can attest that he makes a darn good one, but he is always tweaking the recipe to find the ultimate guac. Rick has tried a raft of different spices (salt is essential), lime juice versus lemon juice, different amounts of chili peppers, and even unusual additions like corn and edamame. His bottom line to patients is that all the recipes are quite good as long as Rick doesn't forget to add the avocado (or, in this analogy, the new immune system from the BMT donor).

More patients aren't always better

When consulting with a doctor, patients often ask how many cases of a specific cancer the doctor has treated. Although experience matters, it turns out that the threshold at which it matters most is about five patients getting a specific type of therapy per year. There does not appear to be an advantage to patient numbers higher than that. Perhaps think of it this way. If you were going to choose a restaurant for a special dinner (say a first date or an anniversary), would you pick McDonald's, which prepares the most meals in the world, or an acclaimed small chef-owned restaurant that prepares far fewer? There is certainly nothing wrong with McDonald's—their fries are to die for—but the small restaurant will also produce an outstanding dining experience.

Other considerations

So how does a patient decide on the best place to get treated, particularly if there are some differences, even minor, in what is being recommended? Rick believes that unless there is a new promising treatment being done only through a clinical trial at a limited number of institutions, the decision about where to get treated is likely to come down to nonmedical considerations. Certainly, an important one is who does the patient best connect with. Having trust and confidence in your doctor is important (although probably overrated). But perhaps the most important reason to pick a doctor and institution is convenience for the patient. Rick is a big believer in getting treatment close to home whenever possible, for both ease of access and the proximity of family and friends for support. Rick rarely recommends that a patient from a distant area with a major transplant center travel to Hopkins for their transplant, since most major transplant centers also make darn good guac.

Perhaps unfortunately, insurance also plays a role in the decision about where to get treatment. Check with the oncologist's office to make sure they accept your insurance. That office (and you) should check with your insurance company to make sure it covers care offered by the oncologist. Your insurance policy may cover some conventional treatments but not others.

Cancer terms reconsidered: Words matter

Despite the blight of misinformation available on social media and in today's political discourse, I think we can agree that words matter. I'd like to finish our book by highlighting some common terms and phrases related to cancer that hopefully you will agree from the discussions throughout the book are not always being used quite correctly.

Let's start with (in my best Austrian accent) the expression famously uttered by Arnold Schwarzenegger in the movie *Kindergarten Cop*: "*It's not a tumor*" (figure 11.4). You may or may not have noticed that I rarely use the term "tumor" when discussing cancer in this book. Equating "tumor" with "cancer" is one of Rick's pet peeves. The official definition of "tumor" is "a swelling of a part of the body, generally without inflammation, caused by an abnormal growth of tissue, whether benign or malignant." Every lump, malignant or not, is a tumor. So the term "tumor" gets a bad name; it just means a new lump.

"*We got it early.*" Cancer is never diagnosed early in its course. Rather, this phrase is used to suggest the cancer was localized and had not yet spread, or metastasized. Unfortunately, cancer stem cells can travel around the body from their birth, so most cancers are not localized when diagnosed. There are rare cancers whose migrating cells may not have found a metastatic home outside of their tissue of origin, and those can be cured by surgery. Thus, a surgeon's pronouncement that "we got it early," or the related "I got it all," should be taken with a grain of salt. Because most cancers are not localized

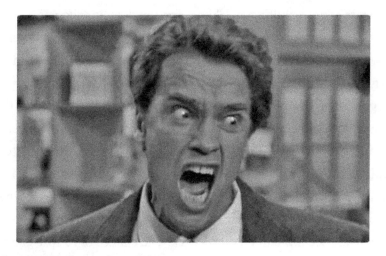

Figure 11.4. It's not a TUMOR.

at diagnosis, the best the surgeon can and should say is "I got all I could see."

"*What do you think caused it?*" As I've discussed throughout the book, most cancers have no cause other than normal cell division. Even for those cancers with a cause, such as a virus or an inherited genetic predisposition, many could not have been prevented and do not produce cancer in everyone. Nonetheless, bad luck can be hard to swallow.

"*Cancer free.*" It is not unusual for both doctors and patients to use this term when reporting the results of routine follow-ups after cancer treatment. However, it is impossible to say that a cancer patient is truly cancer free, since as many as 100 million cancer cells remaining in the body will be undetectable. Rather than "cancer free," the correct term to use is "in remission." Even remission for five years does not always signify cure or cancer free, particularly for slow-growing cancers. In fact, many of the longest survivals are in cancer patients who are not cancer free but cancer controlled. Examples of cancers for which cancer-controlled long survival, rather than cancer-free outcomes, are common are chronic myeloid leukemia (CML), prostate cancer, multiple myeloma, and indolent lymphomas.

"*What are the chances the cancer will come back?*" The answer is always zero, since cancer never actually comes back. Either cancer is gone and will never come back or never completely went away to begin with. The correct question to the doctor is "What are the chances the cancer will relapse?" This is because once the cancer is in remission (that is, it's undetectable or consists of fewer than 100 million cells), it is impossible to say for sure whether every last cancer cell has been eliminated. The only way to know that "weed-be-gone" has eliminated the root (in this case, cancer stem cells) is to watch and see if the weed grows back. The chance of relapse can be estimated, but only in terms of 100 or 1,000 patients, not for one person, who is either 100% cured or 100% not. Even though there may be some unknown, and probably unknowable, factors about the patient and the cancer that might influence the chances of relapse, Rick's answer to this question is to give overall statistics for 100 patients and then to emphasize that he left his crystal ball at home.

"*I beat cancer.*" It is easy to understand this expression of joy and relief when a patient is told that there is no detectable cancer at their five-year checkup after treatment. As much as this term is enthusiastically used and even promoted by the cancer community, Rick despises the phrase. Did cancer beat the patients who succumb to the disease? No, this is not even close to being the case. The biology of the cancer is mostly what determines how successful treatment is, and much of what the patient, family, and doctor do has little effect on outcomes. It can be counterproductive for patients and families to think that outcomes would have been different if only they had tried harder, prayed more, or chosen a different doctor or treatment. I suggest that instead of shouting from the rooftops "I beat cancer" at the five-year visit, shout just as loudly: "I was lucky enough to survive cancer and hold out immense hope that all cancer patients may be as lucky in the near future."

Let's end with a few phrases about cancer that are exactly correct. "*Cancer is a word, not a sentence,*" a quote ascribed to John Diamond, could have been the subtitle for this book. Truer words were never written. "*Don't count the days, make the days count,*" a sentiment attributed to Muhammad Ali, should be the mantra for all cancer patients and their friends and family. And if that is not your mantra, how about "*Not just surviving, thriving.*" Rick and I both hope that our book might help all of us who are dealing with cancer, have had to deal with cancer, or will deal with cancer in the future not just survive, but thrive.

Afterword

CHILL WINTER WINDS ARE BLOWING in mid-January as we await the editorial board's comments following peer reviews of our book. Since turning in our finished manuscript to Hopkins Press in early October, cancer has been "in the house"—our house specifically. Writing this book has been a three-year journey for Rick and me, and in the past year and a half, cancer has affected three people very close to me. As an afterword, I need to share some personal thoughts and feelings on what it has been like living with cancer during this time. In telling these stories, I will both be using the lens of what I have learned about cancer while working with Rick and reflecting on what we have written about it.

Like all experiences with cancer, these three stories are uniquely individual, and for me they are tightly intertwined with love and friendships. First, here are the facts in reverse chronological order. My wife, Ann, always a joyful fountain of energy, suddenly stopped enjoying coffee, pastries, and candy—three of her very favorite things—and died of metastatic ovarian cancer in December within four weeks of diagnosis. My larger-than-life, no-challenge-too-big-to-tackle friend Jack died of adenoid cystic carcinoma (ACC) in November after one tough year of surgeries and radiation, eight good years of living with cancer, and one hard year of unsuccessfully trying several targeted therapies to slow ACC's spread in his lungs. My beautiful, smart, and caring friend Jennefer is doing quite well living with kidney cancer. After several tough months of debilitating symptoms in the summer of 2021, she had surgery to remove one kidney and underwent 15 months of Opdivo immunotherapy infusions, which had manageable side effects. Her last MRI showed "no evidence of disease," and plans are to discontinue treatments soon and shift to periodic monitoring. Jennefer recently competed in a tennis tournament and has made plans for international travel in the year to come.

This has all been way too many "WTH" moments in short order. These three cancers have no known hereditary or environmental causes—just bad luck. Can writing a book about cancer be bad luck? I don't think so. One thing I've learned through this project is that it isn't worth spending much time fretting over *why* cancer knocks on any one door. My friends and I are well beyond that magical age of 65 years, when cancer will catch up with many of us along with forgetfulness, stiff joints, and maybe other more serious ailments.

The hardest thing for me to understand and accept in writing this book is that when cancer is diagnosable, it can already be too late to change the outcome. The progress of cancer takes time: the accumulation of many mutations, periods of rest or inactivity, and a final mutation that stops cancer cells from dying and, for some cancers, starts rapid cancer cell reproduction. This process is for the most part unseeable, undiagnosable, and, for some cancers, unchangeable and unalterable when first viewed. So what is one to do?

First of all, stay in the game! It is possible to increase your odds of avoiding, or at least delaying, cancer by following widely accepted medical guidelines for good health (don't smoke, watch your weight, and so on). Why turn away from an edge that could increase your odds of a longer, healthy life? Ann, Jack, and Jennefer all generally had healthy lifestyles, and although this wasn't enough to prevent cancer, I'd like to believe it delayed its onset.

Second, finding cancer earlier could be life changing. With rapid advances in therapies, knowing sooner rather than later could open doors to a longer, higher-quality life with cancer. At least you will have options to consider. The news is overflowing with research advances in early detection of cancers and identification of genetic markers. For example, research by Bert Vogelstein and others at Johns Hopkins has shown that blood tests followed by scans when blood tests are positive are effective in early detection of solid organ cancers including lung and ovarian.

When considering cancer prevention and screenings, what makes sense for any one person comes down to risk assessment and risk tolerance. Simplistically, what are your individual risks for cancer based on family medical history, health, and lifestyle? Is early detection beneficial? Surprisingly, the answer isn't always yes. Are you risk averse (needing to know everything that is knowable as soon as possible), risk tolerant (willing to accept a reasonable amount of risk), or a risk junkie (willing to go with life's flow and all possible outcomes)? One or more expert guides through this thought process and the constantly evolving cancer knowledge base will almost certainly be needed. Find a good guide who will take the time to assess your risks and help you to come up with a plan for cancer prevention and screenings that feels right. There is no one-size-fits-all plan.

With hindsight, Ann had two risk factors for ovarian cancer—no pregnancy and her age (73)—and she should have continued more regular pelvic exams beyond age 66. Medicare covers pelvic exams every 24 months or, for people with high cancer risk, every 12 months. It is possible that a gynecologist could have felt her ovarian cyst earlier and follow-up tests could have been done: a vaginal ultrasound, an ACC blood test for ovarian cancer, and a CT scan. Late diagnosis of ovarian cancer is not uncommon. Ann never felt the 9.8-centimeter (3.8-inch) cyst on her left ovary. Frequent urination was the one telltale symptom, but that didn't show up until very late. Her other symptoms—tiredness and abdominal pain—were also late in appearing and related to her failing liver, where the ovarian cancer had metastasized and was spreading rapidly.

Would earlier diagnosis through a pelvic exam have made a difference in Ann's life expectancy? Probably not soon enough, since there is no cure for ovarian cancer and the path of Ann's disease and liver metastasis would have already been set. At best, earlier chemotherapy might have slowed her liver failure buying her some more time—months, maybe longer; it's impossible to know or predict. Would living an extra year with no hope for a cure, a failing liver, and recurring chemo treatments have been worth it? I don't know what Ann might have decided, but she would have wanted that decision to make. I hope that research into earlier cancer detection matures into best practices that will afford future cancer patients earlier and better choices.

So what have I learned from living with my wife and friends' cancers over the past year and a half?

First, while the fear of the big, unknown, "capital C" cancer of my early years is greatly diminished, the individual experience of cancer, with its many complexities and life-altering decisions, is still frightening. It takes great courage, the loving support of family and friends, and knowledgeable and sensitive guides to navigate these dark, choppy waters.

The second thing I've learned is that you must put on your own oxygen mask first. It is hard meeting your loved one's increasing needs and managing doctor and hospital appointments, drug regimens, medical procedures, and maybe hospitalization. It is easy to get overwhelmed and down. Look out for your core needs: food and sleep.

Third, get help. This is the time to surround yourself with family and friends. Let them take over at times. Ann needed a lot of help in the hospital, and luckily I could sleep over in her room. But there wasn't much sleeping going on, and when our wedding anniversary came during her hospitalization, there wasn't much romance going on. Her sister Paula and I tag-teamed overnights, which was critical. More help isn't always better. Too many people helping can become chaotic and sap precious energy. The CaringBridge website is an excellent resource for keeping everyone informed, which can be a challenge, and for getting help with specific needs.

The fourth thing I learned is about living with cancer. As these three personal stories show, there are lots of ways to live with cancer. Ann was unaware of her advanced cancer until the very end, so most of her life with (undiagnosed) cancer was happy and vigorous, as was her nature. Since treatments for her type of ovarian cancer weren't available, not knowing about her cancer until near the end may have been a good thing, allowing us several carefree years together enjoying retirement. Jack's cancer was diagnosed and treated early, giving him eight years of good quality of life during which he enjoyed his mother's 100th and 101st birthdays and the marriages of his son and daughter. And for Jennefer, the success of checkpoint inhibitors in treating kidney cancer offers her a chance for a cure and life beyond cancer.

And the final lesson is about living with dying. For Ann and Jack, when the cancer reached a certain point, their bodies started shutting down: no appetite, foods not tasting good, trouble swallowing or

holding down food, and pain. This was a challenging time both physically and emotionally. At this transition point, it seems wrong to
stop fighting, but it is time to accept that death is around the corner, to
seek comfort for your loved one, and to spend precious time together.
Ann, of course, was ready to call hospice before we were, but we all
breathed easier as we walked in the door at Hospice of the Chesa-
peake. This was Ann's decision, and although we might have liked
Ann to pursue treatment a little longer, we all accepted her wishes.
Good communication earlier had prepared us for this final conversa-
tion, as did advice from Rick and our nephew Tommy, a newly minted
internal medicine resident. It is a skill to ask the right questions and
to guide someone through the transition from active treatment to
palliative or hospice care. If your oncologist doesn't have this skill,
then seek others who can help—social workers, palliative care pro-
fessionals, social workers, or clergy. I highly recommend a book that
I didn't find soon enough, *Living with Dying: A Complete Guide for
Caregivers*, by Jahnna Beecham and Katie Ortlip.

Through all of this, have I learned to not fear cancer? To be hon-
est, I am more afraid of living badly with cancer than of dying from
it. Thankfully, today I am much more prepared for future cancer journeys, given all that I have learned in working with Rick on this project and all that I have shared with my family and friends through
Ann, Jack, and Jennefer's cancer journeys.

May Ann and Jack rest peacefully, and may Jennefer live a very
long time.

ACKNOWLEDGMENTS

We would like to thank our wives and friends who helped us through this book's journey. We would also like to thank the Johns Hopkins University Press for helping us bring this book to life: Joe Rusko, health and wellness editor; Juliana McCarthy, managing editor; Alena Jones, acquisitions department manager; Adelene Jane Medrano, who added artistic and technical improvements to the many illustrations; freelance copyeditor Heidi Fritschel, who helped polish the text in such a positive way; and Kyle Kretzer, senior production editor, who helped us with the book's final touches.

We would like to especially thank one particular friend, Lauren Small, a gifted author and teacher, who provided extremely helpful guidance. And Rick would like to thank his patients, who have taught him more than they could ever imagine.

ONLINE RESOURCES

Here's a list of trusted organizations and their websites where you can find more information and support on your cancer journey:

American Cancer Society: https://www.cancer.org

American Lung Association: https://www.lung.org

Centers for Disease Control and Prevention: https://www.cdc.gov/cancer

Leukemia & Lymphoma Society: https://www.lls.org

Multiple Myeloma Research Foundation: https://themmrf.org

National Cancer Institute: https://www.cancer.gov/resources-for/patients

National Comprehensive Cancer Network: https://www.nccn.org/patientresources/patient-resources

Pancreatic Cancer Action Network: https://pancan.org

Prostate Cancer Foundation: https://www.pcf.org

Susan G. Komen: https://www.komen.org

REFERENCES

Chapter 1. Cancer's Myths and Mysteries

Hajdu SJ. A note from history: landmarks in history of cancer, Part 2. *Cancer.* 2011;117(12):2811-20.

O'Neill A. Life expectancy in the United States, 1860–2020. Statista. Published June 21, 2022. https://statista.com/statistics/1040079/life-expectancy-united-states-all-time.

US Census Bureau. 2017 National population projections tables. Published 2017, revised October 8, 2021. https://www.census.gov/data/tables/2017/demo/popproj/2017-summary-tables.html.

Arias E, Xu J. United States life tables, 2017. *National Vital Statistics Reports.* 2019;68(7). https://www.cdc.gov/nchs/data/nvsr/nvsr68/nvsr68_07-508.pdf.

Medina, L, Sabo S, Vespa J. *Living longer: historical and projected life expectancy in the United States, 1960 to 2060: population estimates and projections.* US Census Bureau; 2020. https://census.gov/content/dam/Census/library/publications/2020/demo/p25-1145.pdf.

McQuilten ZK et al. Underestimation of myelodysplastic syndrome incidence by cancer registries: results from a population-based Australian data linkage study. *Cancer.* 2014;120(11):1686-94.

Siegel J. US cancer death rate has declined for at least 25 years. Fred Hutch News Service. Published January 10, 2019. https://fredhutch.org/en/news/center-news/2019/01/cancer-death-rate-declines-25-years.html.

Surveillance, Epidemiology, and End Results (SEER) Program, National Cancer Institute. All cancer sites combined: long-term trends in SEER incidence and US mortality rates, 1975–2020. Updated April 19, 2023. https://seer .cancer.gov/statistics-network/explorer/application.html?site=1&data _type=9&graph_type=1&compareBy=rate_type&chk_rate_type_2=2&chk _rate_type_3=3&sex=1&race=1&age_range=1&advopt_precision=1&advopt _show_ci=on&hdn_view=0&advopt_show_apc=on&advopt_display=2.

Chapter 2. Cancer Biology

García MC et al. Potentially preventable deaths among the five leading causes of death—United States, 2010 and 2014. *MMWR Morb Mortal Wkly Rep* 2016;65:1245–1255. doi:10.15585/mmwr.mm6545a1.

Tomasetti C, Li L, Vogelstein B. Stem cell divisions, somatic mutations, cancer etiology, and cancer prevention. *Science*. 2017;355(6331):1330–4. doi:10.1126/science.aaf9011.

International Human Genome Sequencing Consortium. Finishing the euchromatic sequence of the human genome. *Nature*. 2004;431: 931–45.

Saltzberg S. Open questions: how many genes do we have? *BMC Biol*. 2018;16:94–7.

Coffer D. Does the human body replace itself every 7 years? Live Science. Published July 22, 2022. https://livescience.com/33179-does-human -body-replace-cells-seven-years.html.

Dargel C. Can wet hair make you sick? Mayo Clinic Health System. Published September 20, 2022. https://mayoclinichealthsystem.org/hometown -health/speaking-of-health/can-wet-hair-make-you-sick.

Bianconi E et al. An estimation of the number of cells in the human body. *Ann Hum Biol*. 2013;40(6):463–7.

Weinberg R. *The Biology of Cancer*, 2nd ed. Garland Science; 2014.

Dexter A. How many words are in Harry Potter? Word Counter. https:// wordcounter.io/blog/how-many-words-are-in-harry-potter.

Johnston HR, Keats BJB, Sherman SL. Population genetics. In: Pyeritz RE, Korf BR, Grody WW, eds. *Emery and Rimoin's Principles and Practice of Medical Genetics and Genomics*, 7th ed. Elsevier; 2019:359–73.

Lee K. Singapore's founding father thought air conditioning was the secret to his country's success. Vox. Published March 23, 2015. https://vox.com /2015/3/23/8278085/singapore-lee-kuan-yew.

Strait JE. Study uncovers inherited genetic susceptibility across 12 cancer types. Washington University in St. Lous. Published December 22, 2015.

https://source.wustl.edu/2015/12/study-uncovers-inherited-genetic
-susceptibility-across-12-cancer-types/.

Chapter 3. Cancer Stem Cells

Sharrow AC., Ghiaur. G, Jones RJ. Cancer stem cell principles. In: Bast RC,
Markman M, Hawk E, Tsimberidou A-M, Kurzrock R, Anderson KC, eds.
Targeted Therapy in Translational Cancer Research. John Wiley & Sons;
2015:39–46.

National Weather Service. How dangerous is lightning? https://weather.gov
/safety/lightning-odds.

Xie M et al. Age-related cancer mutations associated with clonal hematopoietic expansion. *Nat Med.* 2014;20(12):1472–8.

Chapter 4. Metastasis

Jones RJ et al. Circulating clonotypic B cells in classic Hodgkin lymphoma.
Blood. 2009;113(23):5920–6.

Chen H et al. Transmission of glioblastoma multiforme after bilateral lung
transplantation. *J Clin Oncol.* 2008;26(19):3284–5.

National Cancer Institute. Stress and cancer. Published October 21, 2022.
https://cancer.gov/about-cancer/coping/feelings/stress-fact-sheet.

Chapter 5. Clinical Basics

Coakley D. Denis Burkitt and his contribution to hematology/oncology.
Br J Haematol. 2006;135(1):17–25.

Alberts B et al. The generation of antibody diversity. In: *Molecular Biology of
the Cell,* 4th ed. Garland Science; 2002.

American Society of Clinical Oncology. Stages of cancer. Cancer.Net.
Published February 2021. https://cancer.net/navigating-cancer-care
/diagnosing-cancer/stages-cancer.

Chapter 6. Treatment versus Cure

Therasse P et al. New guidelines to evaluate the response to treatment in solid
tumors. *J Natl Cancer Inst.* 2000;92(3):205–16.

Skipper HE. The effects of chemotherapy on the kinetics of leukemia cell
behavior. *Cancer Res.* 1965;25:1544–50.

Huff CA et al. The paradox of response and survival in cancer therapeutics.
Blood. 2006;107(2):431–4.

Jones RJ, Matsui WH, Smith BD. Cancer stem cells: Are we missing the target?
J Natl Cancer Inst. 2004;96(8):583–5.

Kasamon YL, Jones RJ, Wahl RL. Integrating PET and PET/CT into the risk-adapted therapy of lymphoma. *J Nucl Med*. 2007;Suppl 1:19S–27S.

Chapter 7. Diagnosing Cancer

Johl A et al. Core needle biopsies and surgical excision biopsies in the diagnosis of lymphoma: experience at the Lymph Node Registry Kiel. *Ann Hematol*. 2016;95(8):1281–6.

Chapter 8. Cancer Treatments

Sever R, Brugge JS. Signal transduction in cancer. *Cold Spring Harb Perspect Med*. 2015;5(4):a006098.

Miller DR. A tribute to Sidney Farber: the father of modern chemotherapy. *Br J Haematol*. 2006;134:20–6. doi:10.1111/j.1365-2141.2006.06119.x.

Love RR, Philips J. Oophorectomy for breast cancer: history revisited. *J Natl Cancer Inst*. 2002;94(19):1433–4.

Chena M-C et al. Retinoic acid and cancer treatment. *Biomedicine* (Taipei). 2014;4(4):1–6.

Jones R. Bone marrow transplant: pioneering discovery to curing patients. YouTube. Published April 12, 2019. https://www.youtube.com/watch?v=0BtlLdIWqDs.

Chapter 10. Cancer Prevention II

Centers for Disease Control and Prevention. What are the risk factors for lung cancer? Published October 22, 2022. https://www.cdc.gov/cancer/lung/basic_info/risk_factors.htm#:~:text=In%20the%20United%20States%2C%20cigarette,the%20risk%20for%20lung%20cancer.

LoConte NK et al. Alcohol and cancer: A statement of the American Society of Clinical Oncology. *J Clin Oncol*. 2017;36(1):83–93.

Global BMI Mortality Collaboration. Body-mass index and all-cause mortality: individual-participant-data meta-analysis of 239 prospective studies in four continents. *Lancet*. 2016;388(10046):776–86. doi:10.1016/S0140-6736(16)30175-1.

MacMahon B et al. Coffee and cancer of the pancreas. *N Engl J Med*. 1981;304(11):630–3.

Zhao L-G et al. Coffee drinking and cancer risk: an umbrella review of meta-analyses of observational studies. *BMC Cancer*. 2020;20:101. doi:10.1186/s12885-020-6561-9.

de Martel C et al. Global burden of cancers attributable to infections in 2008: a review and synthetic analysis. *Lancet Oncol*. 2012;13(6):607–15.

Zick SM, Snyder D, Abrams DI. Pros and cons of dietary strategies popular among cancer patients. *Oncology* 2018;32(11):542-7.

New York State Department of Health. Love Canal follow-up health study: mortality community report. Revised May 2017. https://health.ny.gov /environmental/investigations/love_canal/mortality_community_report .htm.

Smith RA et al. Cancer screening in the United States, 2019: a review of current American Cancer Society guidelines and current issues in cancer screening. *CA Cancer J Clin.* 2019;69(3):184-210.

Harding C et al. Breast cancer screening, incidence, and mortality across US counties. *JAMA Intern Med.* 2015;175(9):1483-9.

Jorgenson KJ et al. Breast cancer screening in Denmark: a cohort study of tumor size and overdiagnosis. *Ann Intern Med.* 2017;166(5):313-23.

Chapter 11. How I Learned to Stop Worrying and Not Fear Cancer

Gries KJ et al. Cardiovascular and skeletal muscle health with lifelong exercise. *J Appl Physiol.* 2018;125(5):1636-45.

White MC et al. Age and cancer risk: a potentially modifiable relationship. *Am J Prev Med.* 2014;46(3 Suppl 1):S7-15.

American Cancer Society. Lifetime risk of developing and dying from cancer. Revised January 12, 2023. https://cancer.org/cancer/cancer-basics /lifetime-probability-of-developing-or-dying-from-cancer.html.

National Cancer Institute. Surveillance, Epidemiology, and End Results Program. https://www.seer.cancer.gov.

Gale RP, Lee ML. Do different therapies of AML produce different outcomes? *Leuk Res.* 1990;14(3):207-8.

Afterword

Jacobs D. How inventors' vision for early cancer detection got a $2.1 billion boost. *Dome,* January/February 2022. https://www.hopkinsmedicine.org /news/articles/how-inventors-vision-for-early-cancer-detection-got-a-21 -billion-boost.

INDEX

About the Authors

Dr. Richard J. Jones is currently professor of oncology, medicine, and pathophysiology at Johns Hopkins University. He is also director of the Bone Marrow Transplant Program and co-director of the Hematologic Malignancies Program at the Sidney Kimmel Comprehensive Cancer Center at Johns Hopkins, as well as an associate director of the Cancer Center. Over his nearly 40-year career in cancer research, he has been continuously funded by the National Cancer Institute. He has held numerous national and international leadership positions in the field of cancer, including chair of the Blood and Marrow Transplant Clinical Trials Network and chair of the National Cancer Institute's Cancer Centers Study Section (Subcommittee A).

T. Michael McCormick was schooled in the liberal arts and educational psychology at Bucknell University. He recently retired from a long career in systems and software engineering and information technology management. Currently he is filling his time with beneficial and challenging projects (like this book); volunteering efforts (providing food backpacks to children facing food insecurity in Anne Arundel County, Maryland; helping homeless people seek employment; planting trees and whacking down invasive plants); and new and old interests: music, travel, exercise, learning Spanish, and trying to get more than 10 master points in bridge with Rick.